ACTIVATE YOUR JOY

A Transformative Awakening to Health, Happiness and Success, Including 12 Missions to Design a Life You Love

by Erik Ohlsen

Activate Your Joy
A Transformative Awakening to Health, Happiness and Success,
Including 12 missions to Design a Life You Love

Copyright © 2017 by Erik Ohlsen

ISBN: 978-0-9975202-5-5
Published by StoryScapes
erikohlsen.com
StoryScapes
PO Box 116
Sebastopol, Ca 95473
erik@erikohlsen.com

This book is dedicated to the memory of my beautiful mother, Inés Virginia Lucco.

Thank you for dedicating your life to providing me a healthy home. Thank you for teaching me the values of peace, the love of nature, and the freedom of self-expression. I love you.

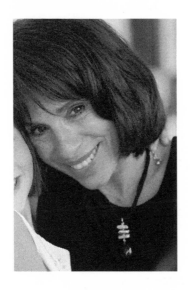

Inés Virginia Lucco
January 20, 1954–August 1, 2008

TABLE OF CONTENTS

DISCLAIMER

This book is not meant to be a substitute for professional advice or support. There are many methods and modalities that can heal the mind and body. This book is rooted in both ancient wisdom teachings and modern approaches to personal development and transformation. I hope this work is as powerful for you as it has been for me, but keep in mind we are all different people and what works for some may be different for others. I would not have been able to experience the powerful healings and limitless thinking without the support of professional healers, mentors, and teachers, some of whom I have mentioned in this book. I hope you enjoy the stories and lessons and have an incredible experience taking these missions. Do it for yourself. You are worth it!

INTRODUCTION

One thing is clear. Everyone WANTS to live a happy life. Isn't that why we work so hard? Why we seek acceptance from others? If we all want to live happy lives, why are so many humans unhappy? Why do we look to the future for a glimpse of happiness? If I get that job, I'll make it in the world. If I find a cure to my illness, I'll finally feel good. If I get married and have children, I'll finally be fulfilled. If I get a degree, I'll fulfill the expectation of others and earn their love. If I change the way others treat me, I will finally have my freedom.

The deeper I look into the emotional baseline of the culture around me, the stronger I feel the collective grief of this world. There is so much suffering, judgment, and victimhood. Regardless of income, race, gender, and culture, too many people are unhappy, unfulfilled, and desperate for a life they love. This collective unhappiness infects the world around us. How do we break the cycle and awaken lives rooted in Joy? Whatever the circumstance, I believe we all have the right to thrive. We all have the right to be happy, dignified, respected, and loved.

How do we get there? Is there even a place to get to? Are we doomed to live in cultures of pain and despair? I don't think so. What if I told you that you don't have to change anything to find the love you deserve? What if I told you everything you need, all the love, support and power you need to live a life to its fullest is available to you right now? You might think it's not possible, this is a scam, there is no way out of your pain and depression. No alternative that you are worthy of. No path to freedom without fighting to the death. But there is ...

You have suffered long enough and it is time to awaken to your life's purpose. It's time to claim your dream. It's time for transformation, for connection, for healing, and regeneration. *Activate Your Joy* is a wakeup call that speaks to your soul. Here, you find the source of love, the transformation of darkness, and the power to create a full and wonderful life. It's simple yet powerful, and the only tools you need are an open heart and a quiet mind. In this book you will learn quick action steps you can take to intentionally design a life aligned with what is best for you. You will awaken the superpowers you already have to create this abundance.

You will learn to master awareness and see only truth around you. Here you activate love, joy, and healing all around you through discovering your capacity for unconditional love of the world. You get to become your own master healer and invite lasting health into your body and mind.

When you use Joy and Love as the frame for living your life, you will experience transformation beyond what may seem possible. You become one with the natural ways of the universe and from there you can harness its power. You will even learn to harness the power of nature and regenerate the community and environment around you. A major reason for writing this book is to remind humanity of its abilities to make peace every day. It starts within each of us.

This book is also a recollection of my own personal healing and awakening to my life's purpose. The writing process itself has been profound as it alerts me constantly to my own awakening of joy and love. Like so many, I've been deep in those dark places of my mind. The places you don't want to tell a single person about. Living a large part of my life experience with a chronic nervous system imbalance, I've experienced tragic loss, depression, anger, regret, and daily discomfort. These are real and intense and over time became a vicious cycle I felt stuck in. It would start with the pain and discomfort of my body and then transform into anxiety, anger, and depression, often in that order. For many years, I succumbed to the narratives that kept me in this vicious cycle, unable to break free from its grip on my mind.

This book is the story of my own struggles and tragedies. Through all my pain, I could still feel love for this world. That love shone through and gave me purpose of a kind. I lived for helping others. I committed myself to seeking justice in our communities and environment. I thought sacrificing myself to these causes was the answer to fill the hole in my heart. I thought the more I sacrificed, the more people would accept me and the more I would feel worthy. When the symptoms of my chronic illness took effect and soon thereafter my mother died, I became lost. I could no longer prioritize the struggles of others over my own personal situation and the emotional paralysis that accompanied it. I was chained to my house and thought I had become worthless.

The funny thing is, my whole journey took me to a place where I never thought I would find answers. Somewhere that didn't even seem a possibility but was always there with me at all times, in every moment. I finally came back to myself. To who I truly am. That is the key to unlocking the most powerful mystery of being human. In this book I will share milestone experiences that have shaped and led me on my path, culminating in the words on these pages.

This book is a re-creation of the rites of passage that have helped me design a dream life, heal and accept my grief, thrive in my relationships, connect with the natural world and experience success in my career. Am I enlightened, always happy, never sad, angry or depressed? Of course not, I am human ...

These very real parts of human existence are important edges for growth and inner transformation. It's the acceptance and surrender of these real feelings that transforms them. It's the awareness and being present in the moment that catalyzes inner power and leads to joy. For me, it's the surrender that allows me to laugh in the face of a coming panic attack or ask for forgiveness when I get angry at my loved ones. The acceptance of what happens leads me to the path of forgiveness and freedom in my mind.

It is a vulnerable feeling to share these stories—some painful, some delightful—and expose all of my growth edges. The beautiful thing is, like in natural ecosystems, the edges are where the most growth and regeneration can take place. Where are your growth edges? Ready to find out? The process outlined in this book is a path to freedom, but it's not the one you think you're taking. There is nothing outside of yourself to learn here. Nothing your body, your mind, and your heart don't know already. My job here is to help remove the mask of stories, assumptions, and attachments keeping you from seeing your own truth.

This book is organized into four strategies for living your life. Vision, connection, transformation, and regeneration: these provide a framework for designing your life, acknowledging your truth, healing your relationships, and growing love and generosity in the world. Each part has three powerful missions for you to complete to activate profound change in your life.

These pages will feed the love that resides in your heart this very moment. This book is here to reflect to you your own capacity for joy. Are you ready? Scared to dive in? What do you have to lose except fear itself? What do you have to lose except the shackles you place on yourself? Enough is enough. You deserve the life you are meant to have. You deserve peace. You deserve health. You deserve to fully be yourself. To be accepted. To be loved. To live in joy. You have the power to give all of this to yourself. In these pages you have a chance to activate all your love and heal the world by healing yourself.

To make your experience even better, claim your interactive bonuses. The *Activate Your Joy Tracking Poster and Life Design Game Playbook* PDF Downloads can be found here:
http://erikohlsen.com/ayj-playbook/

HOW TO USE THIS BOOK

This book is organized into five parts. The first four parts—Vision, Connection, Transformation and Regeneration—are composed of my own life lessons and personal stories. The fifth part of this book is a set of *12 Missions to Design a Life You Love.*

Each of the 12 missions are associated with a chapter in the book. At the end of each chapter you will find a link to the mission related to that chapter.

Feel free to take each mission as you complete a chapter, or you can read through all the chapters first and then dive into the life-design game at the end. You get to choose your own adventure! Find the journey that works best for you.

Don't forget, to get the best results in taking the missions, follow along with your free Activate Your Joy Life Design Game Workbook PDF Download, found here: http://erikohlsen.com/ayj-playbook/

Join the Activate Your Joy Life Design Facebook Community for continued engagement and support.
https://www.facebook.com/groups/184539945414028/

PART ONE:
VISION

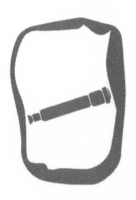

Let your passion paint the world,
Seeds of life you unfurl.
Every moment is your design;
No more fear, you can shine.

CHAPTER 1
THE FRAME OF JOY

*"Keep your thoughts positive because
your thoughts become your words.
Keep your words positive because
your words become your behavior.
Keep your behavior positive because
your behavior becomes your habits.
Keep your habits positive because
your habits become your values.
Keep your values positive because
your values become your destiny."*
—Mahatma Gandhi

Your Frame, The Eyes You See With

To activate your joy, you must first unearth who you truly are. You need ask yourself key questions. These questions uncover the "frame" endlessly running inside your mind. The questions will come soon, but first it's important you understand what your frame is.

In this book, we will use "frame" to mean the lens you see the world through. It involves the stories, life programming, and beliefs that influence your every decision and your every action. For most of us, our frame is the underlying aspect of ourselves that may cover up the inherent love and joy dwelling inside each of us.

The illusions our frames protect are attached so strongly in our minds that we may not recognize their existence. I sure didn't. It's like a program running on automatic in the background, or marionette strings attached to your mind. Your frame is the chief saboteur in your decision-making and drives your default responses to challenging situations and stress. It's the voice in your head telling you "this" and "that" all day long. Telling you that you are not worthy. Telling you what to think, what you have to do, what you can do, what you can't do. Recognize this for what it is. The illusions of your mind may be the greatest limitation you have in life, and you are the only person who can change it. This thought is both scary and ultimately empowering. You have all the power to change your frame and together, inside these pages, we will endeavor to set you free from limited thinking and beliefs.

Until I delved deep into the inner recesses of my mind, I had no idea how much my frame was controlling everything I did. It took many years to uncover my truth, and the revelations have never stopped. Your courage to read this book and complete the missions will quickly awaken you to your own authentic self. I will tell you an exciting secret: you can change your frame at will. Yes, you can. It is easier than it seems and it's the first step to designing a life you love. It's the beginning step on the path to personal freedom.

Identify Your Frame

Changing your frame starts with identifying what is true and what is a lie. All day long we tell ourselves lies. We lie to ourselves about small mundane things and we lie to ourselves about major things. We may tell ourselves we can't accomplish something we have a strong yearning to achieve. We trick ourselves, thinking we know the thoughts and feelings of others through our interpretation of what they say or do. We then take action upon these interpretations, not realizing our point of view is subject to our own personal frame and not a true representation of others.

We judge, and we judge, and we judge some more. We judge ourselves and we judge others. For some people, the judgment is so all-encompassing, so embedded, it leads to a life of distrust. A life of perceived betrayal. Uncovering your frame may lead you to reflect on a number of deep-seated myths about who you are. We will attend to those later in the book. Stay gentle with yourself and avoid judging yourself as we move forward. You got this! Pay attention to the immediate conclusions you make about situations that happen in your life. Check and see if you automatically spin negative, positive or other extreme views about something. Use inner awareness as a tool to discover truth. Cultivating awareness provides the discipline you need to recognize all the lies you tell yourself. The practice of awareness takes time to hone, so stay tuned as we will dive deep into a process to cultivate your awareness in Part Two of this book.

Changing your frame opens up incredible potential for a happy life. What if love, happiness, and honesty became a core part of your life story? How would your life change? What sorts of decisions might you make? What risks might you take? Framing joy activates a whole set of powerful ways of thinking about the world, such as optimism, positivity, giving the benefit of the doubt, forgiveness, acceptance, flexibility, generosity, and compassion. What if your entire life was full of this kind of thinking and framing?

I can tell you exactly what it would be like. I can testify to the process shared with you in these pages because this is my story. I share many of the same struggles that so many people deal with in their personal lives. You may share them too. I have been to dark places, felt lost, unloved, unaccepted. I have felt scared, depressed, anxious and desperate. Changing the way I saw myself and the world was not easy, but it was also the most profound experience of my life. A miracle that is still blossoming inside me. I'm both excited and scared to share my stories with you. They are deeply personal, dramatic and vulnerable. But, I can't think of a better way to share the miracle either. Follow the missions in this book and you will likely experience it for yourself and enjoy your own perfect blossoming.

The Savior Frame

The growing awareness of how my stories and beliefs shaped my view has been no easy task. Each discovery, each recognition, exposed another misperception I carried of the world. This awakening process ignited transformations in my life in tangible and meaningful ways. My relationships, my core emotional patterns and my connection with the natural world emerged, filled with more love, more fun and more beauty.

It hasn't always been that way ...

Since I was a kid, I believed to be worthy of love I had to I sacrifice myself for others. I obsessed over making the people around me happy. I believed my role in life was to fix everything and everybody, but not myself. While I was happy to give all my energy away to others, I did so at the expense of my own physical and emotional health. That's okay though, I would think to myself. I'm not worth much anyway. My worth comes only from how good I am at fixing others.

As a kid, that pattern mainly showed up as wanting to please others, but as I aged and developed friendships and relationships with people, it quickly turned to the desire to "fix" other people. If a friend had a problem or felt sad, I made it my responsibility to help them. I would take it so far that if they didn't get better in the way I wanted them to, I would feel sad and resentful, usually believing a wicked story of my own failure.

Resentment grew inside of me and turned to judgment as I entered post-adolescence. With this new frame of thinking, I began casting judgment on people and things I deemed wrong or bad. Believing in the wickedness of people helped me make sense of a seemingly dark world and my need to fix everything. As my teenage years came to an end, and into my early twenties, I carried a weight full of judgments about other people. I had tapped into the grief I felt for the world (and myself too) and criticized people for their choices. My point of view at the time was if you did anything to hurt the planet or were involved in the economic system in anyway, you were a bad person who needed to change.

My Activism

This belief became so stark I started to project an "us versus them" view of the world. This mentality took many trying and personal transformations to finally begin to allay (many of those stories are revealed in this book). Still, to this day I believe we humans have lost our way. The destruction of the planet, the inequality, violence, and oppression still triggers major grief for the future of humanity and life on planet Earth. The difference now is that I recognize love and compassion as the most powerful tools for healing, rather than anger and judgment. As a young adult however, anger was my go-to power source. I channeled it into activism and traveled the world on a righteous path of the Savior.

Most of my work as an activist was grounded in solutions and so it wasn't all born from anger. Although I speak of this time with disdain for how I framed the world, it is not disdain for the work itself. Many kinds of activist work are founded on love and healing, and history has shown the world changing effects activist movements can make for the better. Make no mistake, for me this work emulated the *Savior Frame* and it felt righteous. This is the view of the Savior, where you know (or imagine you know) what and who needs to be saved. Saviors use their judgment of a situation to identify a problem then empower themselves to fix it. They think they and their allies are the only ones who have correctly diagnosed the problem. Others, who see the situation in a different light may be automatically cast as part of the problem a Savior wants to solve. This was me in a nutshell. I didn't really know it was happening for many years. It made me feel high to live in the *Savior Frame*. I felt my perceived moral authority gave me invincible powers. I was right and nobody could tell me different.

A Turn For The Worse

After many years of projecting this image, something terrible happened. My body rebelled on me. Almost overnight, a chronic nervous system disorder slammed into my life. As a result, my life changed forever. I will go into more detail about the symptoms later in the book, but in short, I have to use the bathroom a lot (every twenty minutes sometimes) and the effect led to an inability to drive in cars and thus I couldn't travel. It was so bad, I even had a hard time getting to the closest town twenty minutes away without stopping for a break. I became essentially bound to the land where I lived. My world turned upside down. What was happening to me? I had no answers and it terrified me. Over a year of varying visits with doctors, healers, acupuncture, herbalism, Feldenkrais, western medicine and so on, I still had not received a diagnosis.

A dark path unfurled in front of me as my symptoms worsened and chronic anxiety set in. One of the most distressing aspects of this time was my relationship to who I believed I was supposed to be. My relationship and world-view was strongly tied to the frame of a Savior. House-bound and unable to travel, how was I supposed to continue my activist work? How was I going to pay for my new medical expenses and rent the place I was living? As an activist, people fundraised for me and donated money to our organizations. This financial support was foundational to meeting my basic needs. Afraid of what I was becoming, I was forced to think about making money in some new way. I felt angry at my body. I constantly asked my body, "Why won't you just work correctly! I'm only twenty-four years old. You are not supposed to do this to me."

You see how my frame of the world was already changing due to my health crisis?

Metamorphosis

I was getting married the next year and had dreams of starting a family. How was I going to make those dreams come true? The path I was on was shifting and I was scared of where it would take me. Luckily, as an optimistic and driven person, I was able to open myself up to the metamorphosis taking place in those first two years of chronic illness. On the heels of this change, I was able to start my first company, an ecological landscape contracting company, and I married the woman of my dreams, my wife Lauren. Unbeknownst to me, my frame was shifting dramatically during this time. The way I saw myself, the world and my relationships evolved into new way of thinking I never thought possible. Just starting a company was a huge emotional mountain I had to climb.

At that time in my life, filled with judgment, I disliked anything to do with the words "business" and I certainly hated money. Having to start a business and make money made me feel like a fraud. I expected all of my friends and allies to turn against me and see me for the fake I was. You see, I always knew I was a fake. The problem with being a Savior is you're so focused on the outer world, you never give justice to the reality of your inner world. This misalignment of the inner world with the outer world festers into deep-seated and unseen resentments. What was I going to do? My strongly held beliefs dissolved under the pressure of an increasingly stressed out body and mind. My sickness burned a major part of the Savior frame out of my system and all that was left was vulnerability and humility. I couldn't give up on life and so I pivoted. I chose to turn my problems into solutions to grow a successful life. I began to accept my reality and build a new life from the ashes of the old as I finally accepted my situation.

The Victim Frame

The *Savior Frame* is not the only lens I saw the world through. The identity as a Victim was also a pervasive underlying story living inside me. I had covered up my Victim story with twisted layers of the Savior story I wanted to believe about myself. I did this intensely; I didn't think the *Victim Frame* could ever survive inside of me.

When I was as a teenager, my beautiful and wonderful mom got very sick. She experienced a life-threatening emergency resulting in surgery. A year later, a chronic illness surfaced in her. She gradually fell into a deep cycle of victimhood stories. It's clear she carried these her whole life to a degree but after her escape from death, the *Victim* identity became the forefront of her thoughts and the driver of her actions. Traumatically for my family, our strong and independent mother used her chronic issues as a manipulation device in her relationships. I was heartbroken. She pushed her friends and family away, becoming more and more alone.

The tragedy of these changes occurring to my mother cannot be understated. She was a powerful, loving, compassionate and driven person. Born in Argentina and moving to the United States at the age of seven, she survived growing up in the barrios of Los Angeles. A proud and self-identified Latina woman, she spoke three languages fluently, raised three children starting at the age of seventeen, and worked her way through nursing school becoming a talented nurse who was respected throughout her career. She loved her children fiercely, and taught us many important ways of the world. She taught us to care and protect other people and the environment. She nourished us with her loving embraces and her unrelenting belief in who we were. She loved being outdoors and was an accomplished rock climber, hiker, and nature enthusiast. She was powerful, playful and funny. She could light up an entire room with her infectious charisma. She was my mother, and I love her dearly.

After she got sick, I would go visit her and did my best to make her smile and show her how loved she was. Sometimes, when my mom was having an emotional meltdown, I would plead with her to acknowledge how loved she was to embrace the support and nurturing my siblings and I strived to give her. While sometimes I felt like we got through and she would lighten up and see the beauty in the world again, these periods did not last long and she would quickly slide back into her pain like a child's security blanket. Nothing I ever did to help my mother seemed to stick.

Victimhood

These were challenging and confusing years in my family. The more my mom made herself a victim, the more I vowed to never be one. I told myself over and over, I would never manipulate the world this way. I will never use my grief and pain as a means to control others. It was certainly an honorable thought to have, but I had not awoken to my true nature yet. Later I would discover just how deeply rooted the *Victim Frame* already was inside me. Now, looking back, I can see the victimhood pattern was playing out in my consciousness all along straight through childhood. Why would someone emulate this way of looking at the world? What is the point of empowering the victim? Is it simply about control and manipulation of others? Revenge? Many folks can probably relate to having someone in your life who acts like my description of my mother or maybe you are noticing your own tendency towards this way of being. What is this pattern really about?

The answer I discovered is so simple and yet complex at the same time. It's the need for love and acceptance from others. For many of us, it is really that clear cut. Without a strong connection to the inner well of love that lives inside us, we can feel disconnected. Alone in the world, an outcast. These beliefs foster a need to seek love and acceptance from others. You know the feeling when something happens to you, maybe you were hurt, or you experienced a traumatic event? Remember what it felt like to have friends and family help you out? Care for you and offer you support? That can be a wonderful feeling and that's the feeling many victims crave all the time. It can become easy to then make a habit of using your pain as a means to get that care and love you desire. As a victim, it can also be hard to ask directly for support. The fear of rejection and the further pain this could cause can be too much to bare. By not reaching out for support, it means only the people who care enough about us will come to our rescue. I felt this myself for long stretches of my life. As a child, I would do the same exact thing. If someone hurt my feelings, I would sulk away. Silently withdrawn, waiting, silently pleading for someone to talk to me.

Once I hooked support and attention from someone, usually my mom or a teacher, I would maintain my sadness, my victimhood, thinking it would make them love me even more. I wanted them to pay attention to me. I wanted them to do things for me, make me feel better. Then I would know I'm worthy. Was this what made me worthy of love?

When my mother got sick, she expressed an even deeper reflection of the victimhood I also unconsciously felt. At that point I made a vow, I would not be a victim any longer. I would not use my pain to control others. I would not manipulate my loved ones to gain their love. Or so I thought at the time. That was when I let the Savior frame take over my life. A teenager with a sick mom and powerful vow. Little did I know I buried a nugget of victimhood deep inside my newfound Savior mentality ...

Uncovering the Truth

Many years later I would uncover the truth. I had used my frame, as well as my love of the world, to earn a fair amount of success in life and manifest my goals. I was still living with a ton of anxiety and was physically unwell but ignored it the best I could. No matter how successful I was at accomplishing my goals, happiness never seemed to stay for long.

Looking back now, I can see I was living a lie. I had found a clever way not to face my own demons. I had convinced myself into believing these new stories while the old story festered inside. This could not last forever. Someday, I would experience a reckoning and face all the old grief, stories, betrayals, and lies I had told myself for so long. When it did come at last, I was shocked to discover the deep-seated Victim story was still running on autopilot in my mind.

This did not come to light until an intense and eye-opening therapy session with my wife and an amazing healer. The truth was reflected to me; I had broken my vow. I was doing the exact same thing my mother had done. Unknowingly, I was using the symptoms of my physical injury and the discomfort I felt as a way to manipulate my family. I was playing the victim and I had no idea.

This was a somewhat complex mind frame I had created. While trying to treat my illness, I had become confused with how to be authentic with myself and still be the Savior. This was where I went wrong. My body and my heart couldn't live in the Savior frame and be healthy simultaneously. All of my pleasing of others was inauthentic because what I really needed was to deeply care for myself. By focusing on pleasing others, I ignored my physical condition and without conscious thought, used the pain it caused me to manipulate the people closest to me, a result of victimhood behavior. I used my discomfort as a means to weasel out of responsibility when I could not follow through on my commitments.

Of course if I had been true to myself, I would never have said yes to all those commitments in the first place. Wait! Being true to myself? Was I allowed to do that? What if being true to myself meant saying no to what others expect of me? What if being true to myself meant letting go of the persona I had created? I would let people down, right? If I did what was true to myself I would have to give up so many of the patterns I worked so hard to achieve. If I really wanted to heal my body and respect my nervous system, then I would need to step away from my work world. Become unavailable to my students and retreat into a healing space. Was that even possible? Wouldn't everything I worked so hard for crumble?

The Courage to Break Free

When I finally broke free from the shackles of my thinking, when I chose truth over story, what I discovered was pure love. Pure, unconditional love. That is what was hiding under the Savior and what was covered up by the Victim. That was not what I expected.

I finally had activated Joy in my life and it came in overwhelming waves of laughter, tears and gratitude. This is the Joy we are activating in this book. I'm going to share with you the exact process I went through to awaken to my life purpose. We will go directly to the source of love and the power of awareness always accessible to you. It is accessible to you in this very moment. The truest love to be found on the planet is the love I give to myself. It's the love you give to yourself too.

Become present to the stories running unchecked inside you. This is the first step to the awareness of who you truly are. Don't judge yourself for what you discover. Instead, accept yourself completely. Surrender to what you find, it is the only way to transform it. Resisting what is will only feed the tension and the stories. It is paradoxical, but it is also the key to transforming your frame completely. Every discomfort you feel, every judgment you make, every time you get angry, you feel you have failed yourself or others, these are the moments of change. These are the moments to fully accept yourself and give yourself the love you crave. This leads to a new frame. A new way of seeing the world. This frame is the lens of Love and of Joy, the truth behind the lies; it will set you free. How exciting, right?

Make Joy Your Mission

As soon as you make Joy your mission, make Joy your frame, your whole approach to life changes drastically. You look for what is joyful in your life rather than subconsciously looking for more pain. You slowly disconnect from painful connections which don't serve who you truly are. With Joy as your mission, you make every major decision within a context of what truly makes you happy. This will guide you in incredible ways. Does this mean you will always be happy in every moment? Nothing can ever make you upset or sad again? No, not at all. You are still a human being living in a world full of lies, pain and grief. The big difference is now you're aware of the beauty and love around you in every moment as well. You are not the lies and pain; they are not you.

After my first real awakening to the joy and love of who I am, it became my addiction. This became a problem of its own. When I would find myself getting upset about something or if I woke up feeling frustrated, I judged myself again. "Erik, why are you feeling and acting this way? You're supposed to be connecting to your happiness, remember? What is wrong with you?" These thought patterns further disconnected me from my happiness. I began to learn what I consider a heightened level of awareness. Accept reality for what it is in the moment. Surrender to What Is. It is so counterintuitive, yet so true at the same time. I could see my resistance to what was increased my discomfort and propelled me further from the happy feeling I was craving.

Accepting The Present

Accepting "What is" aligns me with the present moment and present situation. In the most difficult situations, this kind of surrender leads to incredible solutions. I had to experience this a few times before I could really believe it. I have found my response to a problem is *always* more effective once I surrender to the reality of the moment. Whether it is an oncoming panic attack or a sick child in the middle of the night, the solutions always came after I accepted the situation.

Learning to live in this way of acceptance has aligned my frame of Joy with reality, which is a powerful lens to use to see the world. As a result, I feel less fear and anxiety. This enables laughter, compassion, and a calming sense of being to become more and more accessible to me every day. For the most part, my decisions are now in sync with my happiness. I dwell less on the negativity that is so pervasive throughout our culture. I used to spend sleepless nights churning thoughts over and over, worrying about something someone said or something someone did. Now I can accept whatever happens and take effective action or non-action, whatever is required and allied with my truth.

Once you decide and experience the *Joy Frame*, it becomes easier to make healthy boundaries in a loving way. Like me, you may find yourself awakening to the miracles of this world. You will see how beautiful all the people in your life are, no matter your stories or past with them. You start to see gems of goodness in everyone and everything. You may even find yourself smiling to yourself or laughing out loud at the sheer beauty in everything. You see, your joy connects to the joy in everything, and this creates an incredible relationship with all things. Your ability to recognize the good and to appreciate the wonders of life weave an inextricable harmony between you and the world. With this harmony, miracles happen.

As amazing as it sounds, this kind of magic and beauty are happening to us and around us all of the time, and in every moment. Our level of awareness dictates our level of openness to sense the beauty of this world. If we allow ourselves to be distracted by negative frames of thinking, by our limiting beliefs and the insatiable needs of our egos, we will miss the beauty existing in every moment.

The key to this way of life is both terrifying and liberating. The key is all about you. No longer can you blame others for how you feel. No longer can you expect others to make you happy. To frame Joy means taking *full* responsibility for who you are and what you feel. There can be no other way. The choice is yours and only yours to make.

Take Responsibility for Your Life and Be Free

You are the only person who can truly care for your needs. The love you yearn for, the needs of your body, the decisions that make you happy, are all dependent on you and you alone. Of course, some of us may be privileged to grow up in safe communities with more opportunities than others. Regardless of circumstance however, each and every one of us is still responsible for the actions we take in life. We are still responsible for our own thoughts and our own emotions. We all have the power to affect change inside ourselves for our own sense of happiness. Can you see how empowering it is to take responsibility for yourself? Can you see no matter what situation you find yourself in, what you truly seek to be happy and free is inside not outside of you?

Do you still fight with the reality of the moment? How effective has this been? What if you surrender to the reality of this moment, creating space inside your mind and heart to simply breathe? To smell the fresh air? To enjoy the beautiful patterns of your own skin or the sensation of drinking water? These are simple yet valuable actions to alert you to presence. This presence helps you activate your own power to enjoy your life no matter the situation. Relying on others or the system you live in for your happiness is always doomed to fail. This is another way of wrapping yourself up in stories and illusions. The only real place of influence you have towards a happy life rests with you. Do you want to choose this for yourself?

What does taking responsibility look like? If you live in the frame of Joy, many of your decisions will reflect your happiness. You will find yourself saying yes to opportunities that serve your joy and saying no to situations that don't. It sounds easy but can be extremely difficult. I still have a challenging time saying no to things I know will cause me grief. There is so much pressure from the outside world, from our families, friends, and society. These pressures can confuse our decision-making processes about what to invest our time into. Many times a week and even per day, I feel these external pressures. I'm afraid if I refuse to act on the expectations of others, it will change how they view me. Do you ever feel this way? Do you feel sometimes you are doing and saying things because other people expect something from you? Do you succumb to these pressures even when it goes against your truth?

Signals to Your Truth

How do you know what is even true for you? Deciphering your truth can pose a great challenge. Fortunately, we were all born with an incredible tool to signal truth. The nervous system of the body contributes vital information if you are willing to hear it. Most people have heard the phrase "Trust your gut." This is your body talking and trying to guide you. When you listen to these messages, the action you take can be rewarding and enlightening.

For me, my physical state helps me stay connected to my true nature. I have learned to trust my body and what it tells me. I can feel the anxiety and stress of decisions I need to make. This gives me a powerful indication of what might or might not be aligned with my goals of living joyfully. You don't need to have a chronic illness to use the body as a tool for awareness. We all have this innate sense our bodies provide if we listen to it. It is an effective tool but you will want to be careful, all the same. The body's senses can trick you, depending on your thoughts and emotions. I trip myself up all the time listening to my body as it responds to stories and assumptions I make about people and situations. This is why cultivating a strong practice of inner awareness is so essential.

When is the body signaling truth and when is it responding to stories? How do we make aligned decisions that remain in sync with our true nature? How can I know what my body's reaction is trying to tell me? This will be different for everyone and in this book you will get a full quiver of tools for decision-making and awareness. In the next chapter we will explore the power of creating a clear narrative for yourself and your life. This will help guide you in deciphering what is true for you and what is lie.

When you're ready to see the world with new eyes, take the first mission ...

Mission: Transform Your Frame of Mind
Go to Page 165

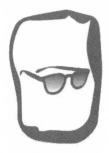

Two Levels
1. Identify Your Current and Ideal Frame
2. Transform Your Frame of Mind

CHAPTER 2
YOUR PERCEIVED LIMITATIONS

"What you think. You become. What you feel.
You attract. What you imagine. You create."
—**Buddha**

You are powerful beyond your beliefs. You may or may not believe it now, but by the end of the book you will be vested in this realization. The deeper this truth roots in your heart, the faster you will make your own dreams come to fruition. Surprisingly, success doesn't come just through hard work, but by letting go of your perceptions. Effort and action is required, but without belief in yourself, you could work yourself senseless and still not succeed in living joyfully. The goal is to work within your own nature rather than against it.

I spoke before about how my frame of mind had changed when my physical condition became challenging and how after being molded and unraveled by my physical discomfort and my mental anxiety, I finally surrendered to my reality. When I did this, I unlocked a key to my own success. I stopped considering myself "a sick person" and began to see myself as a visionary with skills and a solution.

My First Business

I created my first successful business out of this time. I miraculously was hired for a large ecological market garden project only a mile from my house. This project not only gave me the financial sustenance I needed at the time, it also provided an opportunity to be creative, develop a demonstration landscape to show what's possible in an ecological market garden, and hire friends and family to the project. The fact it was only a mile from my house was serendipitous because, as you may remember from my earlier story, I had a hard time traveling long distances. This initial project became the springboard for my entire design and contracting business, later named Permaculture Artisans. Over the next two years I would design and install beautiful and resourceful landscapes, showcasing all the skills and artistic creativity of my team and myself. Not only that, we made tangible restorative changes on the land to support a healthy environment. We created rainwater-harvesting systems, planted hundreds of food producing trees, and created a variety of wildlife habitat enhancements.

I was fortunate enough that my first client was also a successful businesswoman. She supported me through the process of growing my business and mentored me through those first few years. Developing this relationship led to opportunities to use her new landscape as a way to grow my business. We began hosting tours and classes for the community, generating positive word-of-mouth momentum for my business. The next era of my life was upon me. This whole evolution to a successful, purpose-driven business was born out of a belief that I could still do good work in the world despite my physical and mental challenges. I wouldn't be a victim to my sickness. That was me tapping in to the limitless potential of believing in myself. That energy is always there and available to every one of us.

Your Greatest Limitation

You are your only limitation. Your thoughts, beliefs and actions are the greatest limit to what's possible in your life. Have you ever had something in your life that you had a heartfelt yearning to accomplish? Ever had a vision for yourself or the world that seemed so obvious, so necessary, and yet fleeting all the same? Is there a reason you never tried to manifest this vision? Maybe you never tried or gave up entirely? What holds you back? Do you tell yourself how impossible it is? The voice in your head tells you enchanting stories about how you will fail. The world isn't ready. Your friends and family will be mad at you. Nobody is going to like it. You don't have enough time to do it. Something terrible is going to happen before you accomplish it and you shouldn't even try. Someone else is already doing it. Someone else is better at it than you are.

These are the same limiting stories I always told myself as well. It is the same for many of us. The good news is none of those stories are actually true. They are only the perceptions we have about ourselves and the world. They are illusions and you don't have to give them power anymore. Right now you can starve these thoughts of food. Make them disappear! You're the only one who can.

Every big project, every new organization, or new business I ever started began with torrential flows of limited thinking. Often, I would dream of an endeavor for months—or in some cases, years—before I could work through my fear of failure and take action. In the end, everything I have achieved in life happened because I took action in spite of my fear. Even through all the mistakes, success is always around the corner, through effort, perseverance, and most importantly, being okay with what happens.

Becoming Limitless

Limiting beliefs all stem from two basic foundations. The first foundation is fear itself. Fear of what would happen. The risks you would have to take. The outcome, good or bad. Not knowing of the result of taking an action can generate so much fear, we don't even try.

Even deeper than fear is the second foundation of limited thinking, lack of self-love. This is a paradoxical maelstrom of dysfunctional thinking. We starve ourselves of self-generated loving energy, and don't accept ourselves fully. Instead we paradoxically look to others and the world for the love we desperately need. We spend our energy, our life force, in search of acceptance, often discovering disappointment in the end.

That is where the fear stems from. It's the ego-driven mode of living. An obsession with what friends, family, coworkers and the culture think about us. Ultimately, there is only one person who can truly make you happy and give you all the love you need. That person is you. Take the energy you expend striving for love and give it to yourself instead. Accept who you are right now, no matter your current state. This will unlock your potential. Your perceived limitations vanish as you reclaim your own love and your own power. Once you can do this, you unlock limitless potential.

Tap this limitless power. Everything you need is with you already. Take action on realizing your dreams and accept the perceived failures that accompany them. Each failure becomes a stepping-stone. Each step bestows the confidence of learning. Find the courage to take risks. It will turn out better than you think. It may be different. It may take more time. Maybe much more time. But it will always be better than not trying at all.

So many times in the life of my business, I found myself running up against seemingly insurmountable obstacles. Enduring sleepless nights working out solutions to my problems, whether they were with a particular landscape project, a challenging employee, or the fate of the company itself, I had to innovate solutions based on my situation and usually it meant taking risks. Usually it meant having faith in myself and in the universe. Sometimes I would put everything on the line because that was the right thing to do for me at the time. The most challenging times in my business catalyzed successful change only when I was able to let go of my previous ideas and embrace what wanted to emerge.

Fear or Success?

What if success, whatever that means to you, blossoms from your fearless actions? But success can be even more terrifying than failure, can't it? If you succeed, then what? How would people look at you then? How would your life change? Do you really want the change? This thought pattern easily reigns in our minds. Success is never what our mind thinks it to be. Success comes in the effort, not the outcome. It comes in the growth of experimentation. It's the integrity of following your heart and the faith of listening to intuition. It is not wealth and prosperity. It's not the house and the car, the job and the education. Success is following your dreams, no matter what happens. Success is activating Joy in your heart as a mode of living. It's spreading love and generosity throughout your life and others. It's the legacy we find in our hearts when we are on our death beds. The relationships, the contributions, the fearlessness, the creativity, the joy of living our lives. That is the success we are actually striving for. That is the success you can find here and now.

The fact you are reading this book means I have been successful in facing my fears as a writer. The process of creating this book activated all kinds of fearful thoughts in me. Because of this, I've thought many times to abandon the project. I told myself people would hate what I'm sharing. Folks are going think I'm a fake. I had to dig deep into my soul and ask myself why I was writing this book. At the root, I found my true motivations. I'm writing it for my own personal healing, as a documentation of the rites of passage of my life. I'm writing to support all the people in the world who are ripe for this awakening. I'm wrapping up all my love and sharing it across these pages in the hope it will help someone even just a little. Understanding these core goals, I was able to prompt the courage I needed to write and publish this little piece of my soul.

This process is the same always for me. Once I understand the healing nature or core intention of what I'm doing, I transform my fear and take action. It has been a secret to my small success. Sometimes I may not know what I'm doing. I don't always have a plan. Yet I have trust in myself. I have the joy of experimentation and the spark of creativity. I have faith I will learn what I need to learn to be successful. I trust I will get the support I need along the way and I accept the feedback of whatever happens. This leads me to alignment with what is. I distill all the feedback I get and tweak my approach. I shed what's not working and most important of all, I never give up. This is what it is like to live with limitless thinking.

Stop listening to the "can't" thoughts. This is your first and most important step towards debunking your perceived limitations. It important not to believe the "can't" statements of other people as well. With so many of us looking to the outer world for love, we put a great deal of stock into what others think. Remember, they are seeing through their own perspectives and own frames of mind. It is time to get out of your own way. Give yourself the love you deserve. Realize you are limitless. Doing this will lead you towards activating your own special gift. Your superpowers.

Awaken Your Superpower

Every person has their own set of superpowers. These inherent gifts come naturally as a core part of each of us. Do you know what some of your superpowers are?

Some folks know right away, while for others this may seem like a foreign concept. Don't worry if you feel the latter. If you're in the group that feels sure of yourself, you may be surprised upon completion of the *Awaken Your Superpower Mission* in this chapter. How many of your special gifts are hiding in plain sight? Often our greatest gifts are hiding from our conscious mind. We are so identified with the stories in our heads, we tend to take for granted our own brilliance. It's time to wake up your gifts. It's time to use them for your own good and the goodness of the world. By doing this, you activate the potential for a more joyous and fulfilling life.

Intentionally utilize your superpowers in your career, your relationships and your life. If you do this, you will discover the effortless possibility of living a life you love. When you rely on what comes naturally to you, it takes less energy and less effort. You are aligning your actions with your superpowers and this can generate unstoppable momentum in the trajectory of your life path.

Discovering a Power

I remember the first time I discovered I had leadership skills. I was fourteen years old and was on a journey in the wilderness of the Sierra Nevada Mountains of California. I was on a special Outward Bound trip for "troubled kids." After recently experiencing the divorce of my parents, a failure in school, and hanging out with a toxic crowd of kids, I was truly lost. My family was worried about me. I was depressed and angry. After I was suspended from school and my parents discovered some other colorful activities of mine, my family got together and proposed a solution. They asked if would go on a special backpacking trip into the mountains with other troubled kids and mentors. I was exhausted from the emotional roller coaster ride of the last few years and knew I needed a change. It was worth trying and I said yes.

It turned out to be a life-changing rite of passage for me. While living in the wilderness with peers and mentors, I discovered the meaning of real friendship. I attuned to the cycles of the natural world and to the strength and endurance of my body. As I made meaningful connections with people, I found myself drawn to be a supportive role to my peers who were having a difficult time on the journey. Because of this, I spent a lot of the time at the back of the group during hiking forays. I was also inspired to help organizationally for our little community, contributing to meal planning, community fires, latrine digging and the other logistics to keep us all happy.

After the first two weeks of journeying the mountains together, we joined up with ten more groups, each with ten to fifteen kids and three mentors. At this point, the mentors split all the groups up into new groups based on hiking endurance. Before splitting us up, our mentors assessed each individual for our strengths. I was stunned when they told me that based on their assessment, I fit their leadership category. This meant I would be taking the lead for the next week with the most rigorous group of hikers throughout the ten groups. I never considered I had leadership skills. I didn't even know what that was. It happened to be an inherent gift arising naturally out of the process of living with my peers in the wilderness.

What are Your Special Gifts?

At this point, you may remember a time when you discovered one of your special gifts. You also might be wondering how to discover more of these powers. That is what the *Awaken Your Superpower Mission* is all about, but I want to give you some tools you can use before you start the mission. A superpower is something you can do with little effort but do well anyway. It is rooted in your passion and inherent gifts.

We need to make a distinction between talents you have rooted in passion versus the talent you have rooted in years of hard work and determination. These are also special gifts, and they are all your superpowers, but here we want to focus on what comes from your passions. From your passion we can quickly activate your joy. Remember, our goal is about generating happiness, not overwork or stressful effort. As you contemplate your superpower, I encourage you to feel more than think about your powers. Identifying your superpower is not so much about thinking and analyzing, as it is about intuition. Use less of your brain and more of your gut for this.

Your gut is actually a brain inside your belly. There's a reason for phrases like "my gut feeling" or "go with your gut." The body's enteric nervous system, or "second brain" as it is called sometimes, provides an intuitive sense of what may or may not be beneficial for you. Connected by hundreds of millions of neurons, this network of connections may do more than manage our digestion with its direct connection to the brainstem which influences heart rate and respiration. These gut intuitions are better attuned to subtle energy than the brain in your head. Do you follow these feelings? One reason why we don't listen to our gut feeling is the rising fear we feel when we realize our gut and our mind are telling us two different stories. Most of the time, we go with the illusions the mind has fed us, rather than the subtle truths signaled to us by our "second brain."

Activate Your Superpowers

As a teacher and mentor to hundreds of folks over the years, I have noticed a pattern with many people. Most people use their superpowers only in special situations or with certain people. I've met master artists who never share their art with anyone (not that there is anything wrong with that). Incredible communicators who never identified communication as a special skill set. Passionate cooks who hardly ever cook and so on. Many folks see their superpowers as only hobbies but nothing special. I can understand why people don't use their superpowers to build careers and express their creativity. It is scary to be that powerful. Much of the time we bend to the will of our beliefs or the pressures of family or the culture at large.

For a long time, I held back from expressing my passions. I was afraid of being judged by others. I was afraid to be vulnerable and show my raw and true nature. This was a deeply rooted belief system holding me back. It was all made up in my mind. The truth is, it is scary to express yourself. It is scary to use your gifts in all facets of your life. It changes the world around you, it evokes a sense of great responsibility.

At some point, you have to ask yourself: what is the worst that could happen if you express your true nature? Can it be any worse than living in violation to yourself? Can it be any worse than suppressing the special gifts that you have, thinking that's what others want? I started to ask myself these questions and eventually decided that life is hard living a lie. Why not live my truth and share my gifts with the world instead? The more I did this, the more wonderful my life became. I learned that rather than judgment, people around me expressed gratitude when witnessing my truth, my passions and the sharing of my gifts.

Align your true nature, your gifts, and your happiness with what you do. Your actions will become more efficient. You will feel more joy and find the capacity to share more of your love with others. You will smile and feel accomplished with less stress. I believe the more people express their passions and use their superpowers every day, the better we can heal the wounds of our world.

A Bold Vision

One of my superpowers has always been thinking outside the box. I'm constantly coming up with ideas and visions, even if they don't seem possible. This part of my default state of thinking, this way of being, has always been both a blessing and a curse. The motivation of my envisioning is born out of a sense of dissatisfaction with the state of the world and a desire to solve problems. I've always been in touch with the grief in my life and in my community, and naturally driven to be an agent of positive change. When you're committed to this kind of work, you quickly realize the need to have alternative visions to the problems you are trying to solve. To have a vision for yourself and your life is to intentionally work toward clearly set goals. It's the courage to invest yourself in your dreams. To believe your dream is possible and take action.

A bold vision can be applied and utilized at any scale such as project you undertake, a business you start, or your very own life path.

As you start to develop a bold vision for yourself, I encourage you to think larger than these times. Longer than your life and greater than anyone may think possible. Consider what your heart wants to do. Push your edges and vision to a level that seems beyond you at this time and profound life changes can happen quickly. What seems impossible today might be within reach in a year from now or sooner. Maybe it is in reach in five years or twenty years. The time it takes to manifest a vision is not the issue. The issue is the potency or greatness of your vision. Greatness is, of course, subject to the point of view of each person. For some, a bold vision is healing a long-term illness, for others it may be mastering a new skill.

Permaculture Design Principle

I like to draw on a principle from the discipline of Permaculture Design here. Permaculture is a design science that integrates the basic needs of human settlement—food, water, energy and shelter—with the ecological needs of the environment. It is an incredible framework of principles based on the how natural systems flow and function. These natural patterns, and the functions they provide, are utilized in permaculture to design human and ecological systems. The late and brilliant Bill Mollison, co-founder of the Permaculture Design concept, describes one of the principles in permaculture this way: "The Yield of a system is limited only by the creativity and imagination of the designer." The same can be said for developing a bold vision for your life. Your creativity and imagination are your greatest limits. Don't let fear get in your way. You get to choose to unleash yourself or not.

Welcome to Possible

As I always tell my students, "The question is not whether a vision is possible, but when is it possible." This notion drives home the idea that all visions or changes in a system happen at the right time. Meaning the conditions have to be right before a change can happen. It just won't shift until conditions are ripe for shifting. I must note, even with all I have written here, all visions and their conceptualized pathways are only stories we make up. We experience the reality of what is needed by taking action and responding to feedback. The true path to manifestation then unveils itself. Don't let other people's limited thinking hold you back. Time is irrelevant so don't make the mistake of giving up because something didn't happen in the time frame you thought it would.

Accept feedback and continue to adapt to the changing environment, the change happening inside of you and the reality of the moment. We live on a world full of miracles—natural miracles, technological miracles, spiritual miracles. So much of what we take for granted in our human world came from some person's bold vision, plus trial and error. There are many recorded paradigm shifts throughout our histories and they all point to one thing.

The world is always going to be more beautiful, complex, magical and sacred than we can understand with our minds. One era will always be succeeded by another. The potential for change comes from both our ability to accept it and to vision something better. What will the next paradigm shift teach us? This kind of limitless thinking infuses your visioning process with divine energy. Your actions leave room for magic. The same magic feeding the evolving universe.

To use your inherent gifts to their full potential, take the second mission ...

Mission: Awaken Your Superpower
Go to Page 169

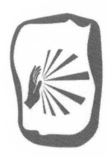

Three Levels
1. Power your Passions
2. Distill You Superpowers
3. Superpower Activation

CHAPTER 3
A DREAM LIFE BY DESIGN

"Your vision will become clear only when you look into your heart.
Who looks outside, dreams; who looks inside, awakens."
—Carl Young

The Ten-Year Plan

For the first time, at the age of thirty-five, I completed a ten-year plan. Many changes happened that I didn't plan for, and in the end, aspects of my evolution were completely out of my control. Astonishingly, the most important aspects of my ten-year plan, the boldest parts of my vision, were intact.

Let's go back to the twenty-five-year-old Erik and the process that initiated this major goal-setting occurrence.

I'd fallen in love and my life was rapidly changing. Although I didn't fully believe in marriage when I first met Lauren (due to my parents' divorce), I could see I had met the woman I was meant to build a life with. For me, marriage is about the sacred ritual and intention setting. It's about a soulful and heartfelt union to build the world together and take loving care of each other.

The Marriage Proposal

Ready for the next phase of my life, I was moved to action by this dream. After a few months, I started planning the marriage proposal and knew I wanted make it a powerful ritual. I made my plan and strategically I decided to propose to her as a celebration of her birthday. It was a few days after her actual birthday and we took a rafting trip down the river near her home. After a thirty-minute cuddle, floating down the river, we landed on a secluded gravelly bank. We got out of the raft to sit peacefully next to the water. I told her I wanted to do a ritual with her but I didn't tell her what it was about. I asked her to trust me and follow along willingly with the process. I kept her in the dark about each step of the ritual so she had to be in the moment. She agreed!

The first task was making crowns for each other out of willow branches we harvested by the river's edge. Weaving the branches together into head-sized circles, we added flowers and other gifts from nature to thread between the branches. We placed our crowns aside and moved to the next phase, building a labyrinth out of rocks. Using softball-sized rocks, we placed them in a spiral pattern large enough for us to walk a few times around before we could meet the center. We took our time to decorate the labyrinth with special rocks we searched out, shells and logs. When we finished I could see the stage was set ...

We stood together at the entrance of the spiral. I began the guided visioning process I had come up with for the ritual. We started by casting ourselves ten years into the future. The spiral acted like a timeline of sorts. We were about to walk backwards in time and when we reached the center, it would be the present moment. Standing at the entrance was standing at the ten year in the future mark. I asked the first question.

Walking Our Vision

In ten years from now, what would your ideal life look like? What would you be doing? What would you have accomplished? She began to share what I knew to be a shared vision. As we walked farther into the center, it was as if we were going back in time towards present-day. Where would be at seven years? Where would we be at year five? The farther we walked into the circle, the closer to the present moment we got. What would life look like two years from now? Six months from now? What about today? We reached the center of the circle. And now, what about this very moment ... Ten years' worth of vision imprinted in the sand behind us. We had walked a spiral. An ancient and scientific shape, a symbol of life, growth, and stability.

Before entering the spiral, we had placed the crowns we made in the center. I motioned for her to pick up this wreath she'd made and I did the same with mine. Then, after commenting on the loveliness of her vision, I began the proposal. I said, "I want to make this beautiful vision manifest. I want to do something here today in this moment to start this new path for us. This is the most powerful action I can think to take." She was glowing and a sly smile formed on her face. I was holding her hands in mine looking into her expectant eyes.

"Will you start this journey with me right now? Will you marry me?" I asked.

She said, "Yes!"

We gave each other the crowns we had made, the first rings to be gifted to one another. After a long embrace in the center of the labyrinth, we walked out together. We honored the vision once again and spoke in more detail about the various phases to make our shared dream come true. This was a deep planning moment and a tangible beginning to our new life together. After spending some time on the riverbank, it was time to go.

A Powerful Magic

On our way back paddling up the river, the wind picked up. Already traveling against the current, we were now going against the wind as well. Struggling through these forces I realized the ritual hadn't ended when we had gotten in the raft. The real struggle to get upriver and back to our car was the next unplanned phase of this ceremony. We had awoken a powerful magic. Working together, we pushed against the current. At times, I jumped into the water pushing us forward while traversing shallow riffles. Was the challenge of moving upriver against wind and current a metaphor for accomplishing our vision together?

Once we wound our way through the strongest currents, we came to a relatively calm area. All of a sudden we heard splashing in front of us. Jumping out of the water all around us were young fish. A sign of abundance. The message was clear. When we work together we get through challenging times and this leads to abundance. When we finally reached the beach where our river trip began, a woman near us called out. She had been observing us and felt compelled to say, "You two look like you're glowing." The magic we had created was so palpable it even rubbed off on people in our general vicinity!

That evening we found ourselves on the coast, sitting on a bunchgrass-covered dune, overlooking breaking waves and a setting sun. We talked at length about our lives. We dreamed, we cried, we shared our gratitude. This further visioning help solidify the ten-year plan we had started making earlier. Our conversations transformed into action plans, timelines, and clearly set goals. The frame of this vision was powerful. We allowed ourselves to venture into a dream-like state that included ideas that didn't seem possible at the time.

A New Narrative

All of this vision was the beginning of a new narrative for our lives together. It was a spell we wove, casting its potential into the universe. That was the greatest goal-setting experience of my life to that point. I was filled with empowerment from that day and it inspired sustained action for years to come. In the excitement of our planning, we never stopped to think about how some of those dreams would be attained. Still young and lacking in experience, it was clear how much we still had to learn. At that point in our lives we were both pretty financially broke and hadn't even started living together yet.

Overwhelming, yet somehow doable. The vision so bold and clear. The narrative sketched out before us like a grand pathway. We both felt a deep knowing that we could make this plan our reality. That's the beauty of giving yourself ten years to plan something. It's like a brilliant, drawn out chess game. Strategic planning over many years grants the opportunity to slowly create a strong foundation for each phase of the plan.

We so often rush ideas and burn ourselves out. Or we give up when we hit our first obstacle or endure our first big failure. We think it is the end when we fail, yet it's actually just a growth edge. An opportunity. Accepting the feedback of failure keeps you on the path towards your goals.

Looking Back

When I turned thirty-five, my wife Lauren and I looked back over the last ten years. We analyzed the successes and the failures of pulling off the vision we had developed. Now blessed with two beautiful children, a home of our own, successful businesses and a generally happy life, we were recalled the specifics of the day of our engagement. We thought about the plans we had made. To our astonishment, we realized every major milestone we had set for ourselves had been accomplished. The planning of that fateful day ten years before had been our north star the whole time. The decisions we made, the risks we took, all worked within the narrative we had created for ourselves. Now is the time to dream the next decade or our lives. A new narrative to be designed, nurtured and manifested.

Now it's your turn to write your own narrative. It's your time to plan a grand path to your dreams. You don't need to have a grand gesture like my marriage proposal. You can do it today with what you learn in the following pages. The outline is here in this book. The tools are living in you, yearning to be awakened, to be honored. The next chapter will outline the narrative goal setting process. *The Design your Life Mission* in Part Five takes it even further. Rise to the challenge and don't be afraid to dream a bold dream.

Developing Your Narrative

Your narrative is your own hero's journey. It's the life story you tell yourself. It is the vision for your life ... One key approach to creating a narrative for your life or business is to start with a non-edited brainstorm. The goal is to use limitless bold visioning to dream a narrative that speaks to your passions. To set life goals that are bigger than you think you can be. If you can dream it, you can make it happen. *The Design Your Life Mission* will guide through the entire process when you're ready but here are some frames to help you prepare for the mission.

What are your greatest aspirations? What is the most beautiful and wonderful life you can imagine? What would you be doing? Who would be in your life? Pay close attention to limited beliefs surfacing during your visioning process. Do you tell yourself it's not possible before even trying? This could never happen to you? These kinds of thought patterns illicit failure before you give any chance for success. The act of intentionally creating a life narrative gives your dreams potential. It gives you a place to start and provides a roadmap towards living a happy and fulfilling life.

Casting Your Vision

The more you cast your vision to the future, creating multi-year goals for yourself, the more inspired you may feel about your vision. Many of the greatest achievements of humankind took many years or even decades to accomplish. Relax into this process and be spacious and realistic with how much time is required to achieve your major milestones. Don't fret as you create a realistic timeframe for accomplishing your goals and you notice it may take years to realize. Always remember, it's the journey that matters, not the goals themselves.

Once we have set our vision, we can "reverse engineer" our way back from our future goals. In this way, we get to see the various layers and conditions that are required for milestones to be reached. This illuminates each step and empowers action to build our lives in real time. This is the recipe for creation. You are your own world creator. You have immense capabilities to create a world you envision. Using the *Design Your Life Mission* found in this book can immensely help you towards clarifying and taking action on your life vision.

For the past twenty years I have put this process into practice with magical and incredible results. You can do the same. It's time to write a new story for yourself. Earlier in this book, we addressed the negative consequences of believing some of the stories we tell ourselves. We talked about present moment awareness and limitless thinking. Get in touch with the story you have for yourself. This includes your dreams, your ambitions, what you think about yourself, what you think about others. Your narrative is the story that you believe about yourself, that you feed and make true every day. What if you designed a new narrative for yourself?

Vision, Story, Action

Turning your visioning process into a new personal narrative is turning vision to story and story to action. What story will you write? How will you show up and be your own hero? Here you can take the time to have intention in the life you are living. To write an effective life narrative, you need to be in touch with your superpowers (your gifts), question your current frame of thinking and tap into your limitless potential. These are foundational tools that help you create a vision in alignment with your true nature. Rooting your narrative in what makes you happy has a tangible effect. It guides your decision making, helps you discover niches in your work, reveals the kind of people you work well with, the kind of environment that supports you and so on.

It can't be emphasized enough how powerful creating a vision for your life is. I have had a number of intentionally designed life plans over the last twenty years with amazing results. Every now and again I need to make tweaks to my planning as conditions in my life change. Expect your personal narrative will change over time as well. The more fluid your plan, the more resilient it will be. If you feel your life narrative falls out of line with who you are, then go back through the steps to find alignment again.

Your written narrative can be formatted in a number of ways. It can be presented as a story, a collage, a mind map, a bullet point list, a timeline or whatever works well for your organizing style. Mind maps have always been a favorite of mine. To learn about what a mind map is go to *Tools of Vision* in the back of this book. Here are some examples of some of my personal narratives over the last twenty years in bullet point format:

Age Nineteen to Twenty-two
- A life in allegiance to the Earth and its people
- Do whatever I can to take care of the planet
- Build as many food gardens as possible
- Organize my community and be a good team player
- Learn to be a good facilitator

Age Twenty-two to Twenty-eight

- Live a life of adventure through travel
- Get paid to teach people about the land
- Take action on the front lines of the movements I serve
- Buy a property to live and farm
- Start a Family
- Start a business

Age Twenty-eight to Present

- Building an ecology of businesses for people and planet
- Spending quality time with my family
- Focusing on my body, spend time every day to heal my body
- Have financial security without killing myself with stress
- Inspire others to awaken to their true nature, support their purpose and direction
- Be a mentor to others
- Spend time in nature every day
- Fill the world with Love

Scaling Your Narrative

The scale of your vision makes a huge difference in the goals you create. In some of my own narratives, I take on a variety of scales from personal to communal. I set goals for restoring the environment and other aspirations of a planetary scope. You don't have to do this for yourself. Scale your plan to what feels right in your heart. What scale of vision is a good fit for you? Let's be clear, we are not talking about fame and fortune, but health and happiness. Not success of things in life but success of loving life. What could it be for you? Follow your passions, listen to your intuition, be gentle with yourself and vision a life that activates your joy.

Your Life Context

Understanding the context of your life situation is an important aspect of creating your life design. Take into account not only the inner world but the outer world as well. Your community, your family, your environment, your culture, your resources and constraints all make up the context of your life. Your frame of mind, superpowers and beliefs also mold your context. Knowing your context helps you align your actions with reality. You stop spinning your wheels, fighting against truth. Utilize your resources and know your stress points. Designing your life is not only about vision and dreaming but also practical thinking, effective planning and efficient action. Awareness of your context gives you a tangible view for executing your next steps but at any point something could happen that changes everything in your life. It could be a new amazing opportunity or a great tragedy. Designing for resilience will enable the flexibility needed to weather whatever life throws at you.

Design for Resilience

It is universally accepted that change is the one true constant. This means that whatever we create is bound to change and keep changing. So why not design our businesses, projects and lives to adapt to change? The ability to adapt to change generates true resiliency. Accepting feedback is a key component of adaptability. Feedback comes in many forms, spoken, physical, emotional, and the better you recognize it the more successful your life will become.

Natural systems provide great models for resiliency. Ever heard the phrase "Don't put all your eggs in one basket?" Nature functions in this way. The functional needs of an environment—its water, food, energy—are never provided by one source or element. Multiple sources for the most basic processes of survival are always in play. This kind of diversity creates a dynamic resilience. The same can be said for how we design our lives and businesses. We can design for resilience by ensuring we have diversity in the structures and processes of our own created systems. Functions like money, health and positive social interaction can all be provided for by more than one source.

A Diversified Business

As it relates to business, I have implemented this notion of Diversity Equals Resilience in a fun and complex way. Ever since I started my first business, Permaculture Artisans, I slowly began starting new enterprises as time, energy and money allowed. A big part of this was following my own creativity and listening to the feedback I was getting in life. Opportunities appear and I pounce on them. But it is not only this dialogue with life that led me to start these various enterprises. I realized early on in my contracting company, I would not be happy being a contractor for very long in my life. It's a stressful business and my body doesn't have a huge tolerance for stress. As I began initiating new endeavors, I saw clearly the decision to diversify my various income streams would allow me to eventually move on from the contracting world. At the time of writing this book that has not happened yet, but this book is part my aligned path for a thriving life.

At this point in my life I own or partially own five different businesses, many of which are still in startup mode. I have already experienced the benefit of having this sort of diversity and "backup plan" in my life and career. A key point of view that I've had to maintain throughout the development of these enterprises is that each one would manifest itself (with my guidance) in its own time. That means I have to come to terms with the fact that it may take years for this diversified business plan to be solidly successful. Who knows, by the time that happens, I may have moved on to other creative aspirations led by my frame of Joy. Life is so exciting this way and this is powerful resilience in action.

Design a bold vision for your life, take the third mission ...

Mission: Design Your Life
Go to Page 173

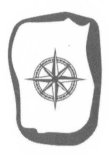

Six Levels

1. Mind Map Your Life
2. Develop Short and Long Term Goals
3. Dream Life Timeline
4. Life Vision Statement
5. Action Plan

PART TWO:
CONNECTION

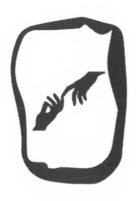

Don't let your pain or your strife
Control all the things in your life.
Get in touch with what's inside—
Your true power, it tries to hide.

CHAPTER 4
CULTIVATING AWARENESS

"Rather than being your thoughts and emotions,
be the awareness behind them."
—Eckhart Tolle

The Most Important Tool

The most important tool you have for transformation is awareness. Your awareness is your power to be present in the moment, deeply listening and at one with yourself and your surroundings. Your awareness gives you an advantage to seeing the truth of things, to seeing the details, the patterns and the subtleties. Awareness comes in different forms. Awareness of our bodies, awareness of our minds, awareness of others, awareness of nature. This is the ability to be alert to what is happening. Not what we think is happening but what is actually occurring.

Many of us live lives that are disconnected from the present moment and thus live our lives immersed in the stories we tell ourselves. The good news is every person has an innate ability towards advanced present moment awareness. It is deep in our DNA and may even be in our souls. Our bodies and minds are made for awareness as well as thought. Can you feel your own presence?

Unfortunately, our modern-day culture often values thinking and intellect over keen awareness. This may be one of the causes of so much of the suffering in humanity. Another reason cultivating awareness is our most important tool for living a life of love.

Take a moment and notice your breath. Notice what you feel inside right now. Look outside and notice the sky, notice the trees, notice the environment you are surrounded by. How often do you observe your surroundings with intention? How often do you notice what you feel inside yourself with intention? This noticing is the first step towards cultivating your awareness powers. As you practice this technique, you may find a whole new world you never paid attention to before. A new world inside and outside of you that has always been there. It is a real world. It's the place you can move with power and grace. In those moments, you connect with the energy of the universe, and that is present moment awareness.

Shifting Awareness

As an ecological designer I have developed an acute ability to observe the outer world. I have always enjoyed spending my time observing patterns in the landscape. The relationship between a tree and its environment is especially awe-inspiring. The way the wind blows through the tree canopy. The birds that land, live and feed from the tree. The leaves and branches the tree drops to the ground to create fertile soil. The fungi that eats those dead branches, popping out of the ground, in so many shapes and colors. If you are extremely aware of your surroundings, you will pick up nuances and important interactions of the world that seem to go unnoticed by most people.

With my outer awareness abilities, I built an entire business, designing landscapes and farms. I used my awareness to create a vocational training school housed at a working farm. I experienced doing what I love and what I thought was the feeling of success. I started a wonderful family and felt loved by them. Even with all this abundance and success, something was way off. I still felt unfulfilled and generally at odds with my true self. I had unhealthy frames of mind running inside me and was blind to key aspects of who I was.

Later I would learn that I was completely identified with my ego and my growing success. I considered my whole identity to be everything outside myself and worked to show my worth to others. The truth was that I was ignoring the persistent inner turmoil, pain, grief and discomfort happening to me. I ignored it so much that even when my body became dysfunctional and my comfort level diminished, I still resisted with everything I could muster. This resistance of reality, resistance of my body, only enhanced the pain. A vicious cycle ensued as I kept resisting. Eventually, that energy turned to anger and anxiety.

Awareness Dissolving Ego

It wasn't until many years after my initial health symptoms that finally my ego began to dissolve and inner awareness began to take root. It was a start to the surrender my body was demanding. Telling me to slow down, telling me to take care of myself in earnest. The ego had to start dying before I could prioritize healing over obsessive doing. The whole frame of my life came into question, and that questioning led to a new beautiful way of being. By listening intently to my body to discover its ailments, my growing inner awareness eventually exposed the realization of chronically clenched muscles in my abdomen and pelvis. This clenching created a vice-like grip in my body, sending shockwaves of stagnant energy into my mind and heart. Prone to anxiety attacks, I had never understood what was happening to me physically. A vicious cycle was taking place as my stress and anxiety would further clench my muscles.

After many years of living like this I finally developed a process for inner listening through meditation, connection with nature, present moment awareness, acceptance, and surrender. These tools help me find inner peace. This peace helps me take responsibility for who I am. Responsibility for my actions, my thoughts and my emotions. No longer do I blame others for grievances in my life. My physical body has become the greatest tool for my developing awareness. When I fall out of alignment with the present moment and anxiety or fear threatens to take me down, or when I'm worried about the about the future or looking for acceptance from others, my body responds immediately. It awakens me to my own disconnection, bringing me home to the present. Home to the truth of what I am.

The Anxiety Vice Grip Cycle

This cycle would often happen like this: when I discover discomfort or anxiety arise and threaten to control me, I first drop in to my inner listening. I then scan through my whole body looking for places where I'm clenching my muscles. I'm always amazed at how much tension I find myself holding throughout my body during my scanning process. I often wonder, am I holding this tenseness all of the time only to relax it when I'm intentionally focusing on it? As I detect these constrictions I am then able to relax them. I calm all the tension I can and what doesn't relax I send my love too. For much of my life I would resist and maybe even become angry at the clenching I couldn't relax, but with my new practice of awareness I now accept it instead. I have even become grateful for it. Amazingly, the acceptance allows the tension to ease just a little bit more. From here, I can get back in touch with that deep well of peace that resides inside myself and every other living thing bringing me back to my true home. My own self-love.

If we want to heal, we have to face who we are. We humans sometimes think that blaming others somehow will release our pain and settle our fear. We blame our circumstances and our situations on others, covering up the truth like a thin scab over a deep wound. The real fear is about allowing us to be who we truly are. What if people don't like who you truly are? How would your life change if you were true to yourself? I'll tell you what it would be, it would be a miracle for this world. For me, I got to experience my own miracle unfold. With attention on my inner landscape, by default, I found connection to joyful living. I found this to be another form of responsibility. Taking responsibility for my own happiness. Taking responsibility for my thoughts, my emotions and my health. This has become the most powerful of practices in my life.

Inner Awareness

Inner awareness is the most important form of awareness you can cultivate to activate your own joy. As you venture deeper to inner awareness, at some point a profound realization can take place. An awakening of your core power and connection to the universe. A realization that you are your only limitation and simultaneously your greatest source of empowerment.

If at the core of your being you find limitless potential, where do these self-imposed limitations come from? They arise from the stories and beliefs you tell yourself each and every day. The thought patterns you have running around in your mind. Remember, many of the thoughts you have are simply thoughts and may or may not be true at all. By cultivating a strong sense of inner awareness, you can use it as a tool to cleanse your mind of limiting beliefs and stories.

But, before you can question your own thoughts, you first must be aware of the voice inside your head generating these stories. Once the voice is acknowledged, you can use your awareness to question it. You can see how much of your energy you are investing in these thought patterns. How emotionally influenced are you by these thoughts? Are they really true? Who would you be if they were not true? When you are deeply aware, you take complete responsibility for yourself and align yourself with the present moment. Once aware and present, you will find a greater capacity for compassion, understanding, and patience.

Sensing Myself

In my own awareness practice, I have experienced a self-observing, questioning, compassion to the Joy cycle. The joy always comes through the end of this process. As I finally sense myself, I sometimes even laugh out loud. I see how silly I am, identifying with this or that thought and I find my center once again. This cycle is a trip back to who I really am. My true nature is always there, under the surface, I just have to be aware enough to sense it.

Meditation, walking, playing music, exercising, playing sports and other artistic activities all have helped turn off the chatter in my mind, and find focus on what I'm doing. This practice of being fully aware without distractions from my mind has shown me the fastest path to personal freedom. Once I experienced it a few times, I became addicted to this new freedom to be who I am. You can do this too!

Start with inner awareness and soon you will cultivate awareness in every facet of your life. Each day will energize you more as your decisions become aligned with who you are. You effortlessly stir up feelings of joy at work, in relationships, and throughout your life.

This connection to present moment unveils solutions to everyday challenges, awakens understanding, strips away falsehood and lays bare the essence of your existence. It illuminates the raw unfiltered energy in everything. Awareness draws your attention to the beauty and abundance around you at all times. It is the absence of obsessive thinking and obsessive doing. The connection to what's real becomes strong as you experience the reality of your life in every moment. You attune to the frequency of other people, situations, and the Earth itself, initiating opportunities for healing, while recognizing love in every moment.

Walk of Connection

My favorite practice for grounding my mind and becoming present is daily walks. No matter what my schedule is, I try to spend at least thirty minutes walking in nature each day. More time is always better, but thirty minutes a day has changed my life. I used to come up with excuses for why I couldn't take walks, meditate, do yoga or some other calming exercise each day. I'm always too busy, the weather is poor, and so on. I would tell myself it would be wasted, unproductive time and staying productive was always the most important thing to me.

The truth is, when I spend time each day centering myself in connection to nature and the universe, I become clear and inspired. This leads to a more enjoyable and successful time. In truth, taking time to ground myself makes me productive! I look back at all those years spent shirking relaxation as unproductive and stressing myself out by overworking. I was just spinning my wheels, feeling resentful about life when I could have been calmer and more capable. A remarkable discovery indeed.

My daily walks grant me space from other people, work, and parenting, giving me the perspective I need to stay grounded when life gets difficult. Without this space, I find that it's more difficult to let go of my attachment to stories and my own unrelenting thoughts. Of course, any time you spend grounding yourself will have this affect. Meditation, running, Tai Chi, all of these and many other practices will get you there. For much of life I always felt I was too busy to integrate a calming practice into my life. I had to acknowledge I was spending my time doing many activities that didn't serve me, rather than prioritizing what actually nourished my well-being.

Grounding Energy from Nature

For me, nature is my best conduit for connection. I use my outer awareness, listening to birds, observing wildlife, and smelling blossoms. I bask in the feeling of air on my cheek and the rays of sun or shade of clouds overhead. This connection with nature reminds me of my inner nature and leads me to inner peace and present moment awareness. Some days it's difficult to be present and it can take up to twenty minutes to calm down. Other days it can be within the few minutes. Most of the time I walk a few miles around a loop trail at the local park. The trail meanders a creek and flood plain, drastically changing from season to season. Filled with willows, oak trees and water-loving bunch grasses, this landscape has been a great teacher.

I've noticed a specific pattern to when inner peace reveals itself on these walks. I may arrive to the park feeling stressed, or anxious about needing to accomplish endless tasks. By default, I tend to resist those tense feelings and subsequently get angry at myself for not being more present during this sacred walk time. A familiar and vicious cycle. What I observe, especially on challenging days, is I become present at the same part of the trail each time. At approximately a half-mile in or fifteen to twenty minutes' worth of slow wandering, a shift in my mental state occurs. The pattern is noticeable, as I finally sense the trees and grasses clearly. As I come to awareness, the environment around me clarifies to a crisp detailed view. I see the patterns on bark, a broken branch here, a blackberry vine there. It's as if I awoke from a dream to never-ending beauty of the world again, always to be forgotten and rediscovered each time. Such is the way of the human mind.

These experiences remind me how valuable a twenty-minute calming practice is. Whether it's yoga, meditation, or a walk, give yourself a minimum of twenty minutes per day to drop into present moment consciousness. Scan your body, accept your emotions and revel in your sacred connection with yourself and the world.

Awaken the present moment, and take the fourth mission ...

Mission: Cultivate Your Awareness Power
Go to Page 179

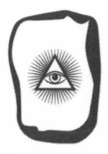

Three Levels

1. Initiate Inner Peace
2. Create Your Calming Practice
3. Claim Awareness Power

CHAPTER 5

THE EMOTIONAL POLLINATOR

"Before you speak, let your words pass through three gates.
At the first gate, ask yourself, "Is it true?"
At the second ask, "Is it necessary?"
At the third gate ask, "Is it kind?"
—Sufi saying

You, The Emotional Pollinator

In nature, pollinators like insects and birds move pollen from plant to plant. The movement of pollen results in glorious expressions of life: flowers, fruits, and nuts, all of unimaginable shapes, sizes and colors.

Every person is a pollinator too, except instead of moving around pollen, we spread emotional energy. We are emotional pollinators. Our behaviors, attitudes and actions leave energetic traces in the people who surround us. All day long, people share their emotional pollen with us and we share ours with them. Think about this for a moment. Have you ever been in a situation where you started the day out with a specific mood? Maybe you felt happy and empowered, stress-free?

At some point in the day something changes, right? A conversation, a message, a trigger of some kind? All of a sudden, your entire energy field changes. Your stress-free mood turns stressful. Rather than empowered, now you're doubtful. Drastic changes from inner peace to anxiety in a matter of minutes. What happened? Energy always moves both ways in nature and in humans as well. Two processes may have taken place when you felt triggered and your mood changed. First off, you were bombarded by emotional energy from somewhere. Maybe another person, the media, or your own thought patterns. Fielding the negative emotions of others is challenging and tiring. Depending on who is around you, it can be like the weathering of a coastal bluff from the changing tides of the sea.

Sticky Emotional Pollen

Most of the time that energy sticks to us in some way. We allow some of the emotional pollen to get through. As always, we translate this energy in our own way, shaping it with our default frame of mind. Realize, right now you have a choice. You can allow other people's emotions to transform your own, or you can listen with compassion to them, grounded in your own well of love and awareness. You don't need to make their emotions your own but you can give the gift of listening. The gift of empathy. You can allow others to have their own journey without identifying with it. When you learn to do this regularly, you set yourself free.

I know this truth all too well. Like many of us, I grew up in a home filled with intense emotions. There was always deep love but also deep pain. A lot of the love and the pain came from my wonderful mother. While she was a bright source of inspiration, love and compassion, sadly she carried heavy grief as well and allowed that energy to dominate her frame of mind. For many years she endured the battle of her own mental and emotional state. Later in life she was diagnosed with borderline personality disorder.

At some point, she began to sling her negative emotions on many who were close to her. I remember near the end of her life I had to be increasingly aware of how much of my mom's energy I would allow to stick to me. She had become filled with anxiety and that scared me to my core. I allowed her stories to go deep into my own frame of mind. I would have to ask myself, do I believe these stories she telling me about herself? Does she really believe those things? Is there anything I can do to help her? Often, failing to help her invoked my own periods of intense sadness and anger, feeling the futility of my efforts.

Spreading Emotional Pain

For many years I could not separate my mother's emotional experiences from my own. With the *Savior Frame* working overtime, I took on the effort of trying to be my mother's cheerleader. I made every attempt

I could to make her feel joyful. To shake her out of her darkness. To conjure hope and inspire her to adopt healthy habits. I made it my mission to make her smile and to laugh. My mistake was not protecting my own emotional body. I was so worried about my mother; I was unaware of the extent her anxiety was infiltrating my mind each visit. I would carry that emotional pain with me, unknowingly spreading it to my wife and friends. At times, I would even blame them for the contention, not realizing I was the dominant emotional pollinator.

Without inner strength and self-acceptance, we keep ourselves susceptible to the projections of others. Like blooming flowers awaiting pollinators, we allow the negative emotions of others to fertilize our minds with their stories. Present moment awareness, a positive frame of mind, a connection to your superpowers, compassion for others—these tools of transformation and protection enable you to choose what kinds of emotions you let stick to you and which kinds you don't.

This is not to say emotions like fear, anger, grief, resentment, and envy are wrong or should be ignored. These emotions are real and require validation, compassion and acceptance to release the grip they can hold on you. Of course, the negative emotions of others will still affect us when we lose connection with the present moment and our own self-love.

Yes, we will feel these emotions too. The key to living a joyful life is not the absence of these feelings, which makes us human. It's the acceptance of them. It's the obsession and attachments to negative emotions that causes such pain. We think resistance is the answer, and we fight the feelings, when in fact, the opposite is true. Acceptance is the real medicine for emotional transformation. Acceptance is a powerful tool I will share more on later.

Harness The Pollen of Love

Luckily the world isn't filled with only negative emotions. There is also good news to being an emotional pollinator. Great, world-changing news! We can harness this social gift and spread joy and love into the world as our pollen. Positive emotions can spread just as fast as negative ones.

Consider for a moment what kind of emotional pollinator you generally are. Are you spreading positive or negative emotional pollen into the world? What words do you use when talking to others? What kind of energy flourishes in the wake of your interactions?

You have the power to heal yourself, and therefore the world, by the emotional energy you share. It is truly awe-inspiring what we can do with this energy. Every person can spread goodness. Spread love to your family. Share joy with your community and bask in the return of that pollen. Emotional energy builds on itself, the more love and joy spread into the world, the more will grow and multiply. Embrace the emotional pollinator that you are. Harness your power to activate joy and turn it onto the world.

Attentive Listening

Awareness of others is key to cultivating a joyful life. Your family, your friends, people you meet throughout the day, your coworkers, every person you come in contact with can affect you in some emotional way. We have to be careful how we bring our awareness to relationships, as we can easily be thrown off track into spiraling thought patterns. Thoughts that pollute our relationships.

Attentive and empathetic listening is a powerful practice that instantly brings your awareness to other people in a genuine way. You intentionally focus your senses to listening to another person. To achieve this level of concentration, you must first quiet your mind. To be fully aware of another person's words, emotions, and body language, you must be intensely alert. Often, if you're able to pay attention in this way, you'll notice subtleties in another person that might generate compassion and understanding, or provide you with an enlightened sense of what may be happening for someone.

Next time you're having a conversation with someone, check yourself on a couple things. First off, are you actually listening to what they're saying? Or did you pick up a few words and you're now developing a response in your head while they're still talking? Develop a practice where you sense what's happening inside your own mind. Catch yourself when you are stuck thinking and not listening in conversations. The speaker will generally sense when you are just waiting to speak rather than being present and listening. What happens when you are able to fully listen? First off, you won't have to make as many assumptions about what the other person said and can therefore respond with more authenticity and effectiveness.

Truly Listen

Sometimes, even in our long-term, close relationships, we don't hear each other. When you finally show up to really listen, you may find out something you thought you knew is completely false. A story you carried around may be dispelled instantly just by attentive listening. When we are always waiting for our turn to speak, rather than listening intently, we almost always respond to a story we made up rather than what is actually being communicated. So many of us seem to suffer from the illusion that we can read each other's minds rather than listen to each other's truths. We must think we are mind readers!

Play around with this a little bit with your friends and family. See if you can discover when you start forming your response to someone before they stop talking. See how it's different when you allow someone to speak all the way through, while hanging onto their words and their body language. Take a moment to pause and process everything you heard before you respond. Ask clarifying questions to gain a full picture of what it is being shared with you.

Of course, it will never be the full picture because they are also speaking from their own perspective (their frame) and you're translating what they're saying from your perspective. Anything anyone tells us is always going through a set of filters, which can cloud the truth. Be aware of this, especially if you find yourself rising in anger or feeling the need to defend yourself. Maybe it is all just another mistranslation, another lie you tell yourself.

Don't Take It Personally

Just because someone is saying something that triggers you, doesn't mean that it's true. You have the choice to believe it or not, but be careful about trying to get others to believe what you think is the truth. With a strong sense of awareness, you should be able to sense when another person is not able to listen you and speaks from their own stories. That's okay, forgive them for their humanness.

One of the greatest gifts we can give another person is attentive and empathetic listening. It is a rare experience indeed to be heard in this way. The practice can be difficult, yet rewarding. I struggle with this practice myself as I still sometimes think I'm a mind reader. Luckily, every day I get practice with my family, friends and coworkers. There is a scale of attentiveness I experience. Sometimes I'm present enough to hear the other person fully but not grounded enough to not take offense when the conversation is emotional. That is because while I may be listening intently to the other person, I am not listening to myself very well and allowing myself to take things personally.

That is why the combination of inner awareness and acceptance along with outer attentiveness and empathy can be an expression of unconditional love. In this way, you can give both the gift of attention to another and stay true to yourself. You allow other people to be who they are and accept them for that. You can hear what they have to say, and share empathetically with them without having to agree or believe what is being said. They are allowed their own process and to be heard completely.

A Tool for Cultural Healing

This listening tool is not limited to one-on-one, personal relationships. As a professional tool for building coalitions and partnerships, working with coworkers, and satisfying clients, attentive listening will unlock many doors in your relationships. If everyone lived and communicated like this, I believe we would have peace on Earth. Shining a light on the truth and growing compassion everywhere ... Communicate with attentive listening and watch your world expand. Take the opportunities healthy relationships will grant you and fulfill your dreams.

The combination of attentive listening with not taking things personally gives you the freedom to not attach yourself and take on the emotions of other people. This also helps you stay clear of making assumptions and participating in distracted communication with others. Grow a keen awareness of your own thought patterns to enable you to catch yourself from forming responses before someone is done communicating. Just knowing what your established communication patterns are will help you transform them. Do this and your relationships will flourish. Your stories of others will diminish and you will find yourself in greater harmony with your family, friends, coworkers and community.

Validating

As a parent to young children, I get lots of practice in dealing with emotional energy. It could be the emotional energy of my children when they don't get along. It could be the feelings that well up inside of me when one of my children stops listening to me. Being a parent is like taking a master level course in communication and emotional turmoil. I wish I could say I was always in control of my emotions around my children. If I was able to do that all the time I might not be human.

There is a skill I use with my children that I find immensely effective. It is a process for validating yourself and someone else. It starts with taking responsibility for my own feelings. Whatever is happening, whatever the emotions are that I'm feeling, it's nobody's fault but mine. That still doesn't mean I won't lose my patience and get angry or project on others. This is why the practice of validation has become so important to my parenting.

The validation doesn't come just by me validating their feelings. It also rests in the validation of my own feelings. Here's how this works using my children as an example. I learned this process for emotional situations with my daughter. She may be upset for good reason, as in a fight with her brother, or maybe it is a tantrum stemming come from something that seems silly, like the cucumbers being cut differently than she wanted them. In either case, the same validation process is applied. Even when a situation seems to call for logic, if emotions are triggered, I've discovered logic will not resolve the problem initially.

Only listening can solve the problem. Only acknowledgment of what someone is feeling makes true resolution possible. Often when I'm validating my child, I ask them simple questions about what is happening. I may ask, "The cucumbers weren't cut to your liking?" Not saying this in a laughing manner, although sometimes it may be hard not to laugh, but to truly acknowledge whatever feelings the child is having, no matter how silly it may seem to me. This validation takes some of the charge out of the situation. My daughter knows I'm listening to what's happening with her.

Validation First, Logic Second

In a situation like this, bringing logic into the equation may feed the tantrum. If I said, "Honey the cucumbers are going to taste the same no matter how they are cut!" She may hold on to her perception of the situation and this likely could escalate the tantrum. Are the cucumbers actually the problem? Of course not! That is why it is so important to validate emotions. It may be she had a hard day at school and can't put it into words. Maybe she's tired, maybe she's getting sick. In the end, it doesn't actually matter what the reason is. It's the process of listening and validating that is essential.

It is easy to use parenting as an example for validation. The truth is, the need for validation goes way beyond parenting. Every relationship, community, and culture could find healing through validation. Often when people communicate with each other, they are quick to make assumptions, invent stories and turn to defensiveness. Without being validated and grounded in the truth of who we are, we become lost. Our identity with our own egos makes it hard to hear the truth in others and in ourselves. Thus, our emotional bodies can be taken over by our egos and result in a quick jump to negative reactions when problems arise.

With all this happening in daily communication with each other, we hardly ever validate one another. When you don't feel validated, you don't feel heard. You don't feel understood. This causes frustration and feeds the vicious cycles of miscommunication. Learn to validate the people in your life. Don't let your ego get in the way. Ground yourself in your own capacity for self-love and confidence. This will lead to a compassionate space to ease the giving of validation to one another. By setting this example for your family and community, others will follow your lead and the healing will spread like a wildfire of empathy.

Accept and Integrate Feedback

Accepting feedback can be one of the most difficult parts of being human. Without doing the inner work to find peace, to focus on happiness, and to trust yourself, receiving feedback from others can be scary and sometimes devastating. Grief is caused by our attachments to what we want, our attachments to our stories, to how we think the world should be. In this fragile state we can act negatively when somebody tells us were wrong, we made a mistake or aren't good enough.

What people say to you, especially when it's critical or providing feedback, can actually be the greatest gift to receive. A gift helping you design and manifest your bold vision. As an individual, you only see the world through one point of view. Your own point of view. If you only allow yourself one point of view, you are limiting what's possible. That is why feedback is such a gift. It's the gift of another point of view, other eyes to see the world through. You don't have to believe what someone shares with you. You don't have to take on their stories. But, if you don't at least listen, open your mind and heart to feedback that is being offered to you, you will miss extraordinary opportunities for growth and success.

With a strong sense of inner awareness, what other people say cannot hurt you for long. Without the distraction of those triggering emotions, you can listen for the gems given in the feedback. You can identify the growth edges and integrate them into your life, vision or project. Easy to say but difficult to do, right?

Critical Feedback

In my own life and work, I have been plagued with the challenge of accepting feedback. When I'm expressing my *Savior Frame* of mind, I work hard, desperately trying to do good in the world. This desperation came from my own lack of inner self-confidence. What happens to me if I then receive critical feedback? I put my heart and soul, my sweat, my blood, my tears on the line, thinking I'm doing great work for the world. All of that sacrifice and someone tells me I'm wrong. I failed! I'm not good enough. These are the thoughts that enter my mind. It's like a sword in my heart. But is it really? Is my righteousness so great I can't even receive the gift of feedback?

This played out with some intensity after I wrote my first children's book. I have always been an avid storyteller but this was the first time I tried to write a children's story. I had collaborated with my wife and children for months coming up with the concept and a good story that would both inspire and educate young minds about nature. Once I had the story to what I thought was a good place, I sent it to my editor at the time. I hadn't really given him enough background about this particular book (it was a story about an actual playground at my children's school) and the editor misunderstood my goals.

He thought I wanted to get this book published by a traditional publisher rather than publishing it myself with the community. After a couple of months, he finally got back to me with feedback about my story. I didn't expect the emotions that surged inside of me when I finally read his feedback.

My heart raced and my face flushed. I felt crushed, I felt angry. In short, he thought the story was unfit for publishing and went on to tell me what an inexperienced writer I was. He pointed out critical errors in my story and prompted me to take the next year to research and learn before he thought I could publish a book. I felt like a complete failure and started to worry that my family and friends would also think my story was complete garbage.

This has often been my first response when I receive critical feedback. I'm so identified with all the hard work, I become sensitive to the feedback given. Regardless, whether the editor in this case was being insensitive, or everything he shared with me was the absolute truth, the only thing that really mattered was my response.

Finding The Gifts of Feedback

After a couple days however, I was able to read back through his feedback. Now it didn't seem quite as bad as it did the first time. In fact, he pointed out some major gaps in the story that were crucial to it being understood by readers. His feedback actually changed my whole trajectory for the story as I finally surrendered to the gift of a professional editor's advice. I made major improvements to the content and flow of the book, integrating this feedback.

Ultimately the book turned out to be a wonderful experience and a great success through the lens of accomplishing my first self-published children's book. My children were so excited to see the book finally printed and the community embraced our story of the playground.

This is where the strength of humility aids in our resilience. Do good work, but let's not attach ourselves to the work in such a way that we set our expectations up for failure. There is no failure. Let the righteousness dissolve. Let humility reign. From a humble place we can receive the beauty of feedback. Once feedback has been received the next task is to integrate it. First, let's look at a practices for receiving feedback.

Take Time to Integrate

One trick to accepting feedback is to not respond right away if you feel your emotions begin to rise. I can't say enough about how important it is to take your time to respond to feedback, especially if it initially hits you in a negative way. Responding right away when provoked intensifies the likelihood you say or do something you regret later. A quick response with anger doesn't represent the integrity of who you really are, does it? Take time to consider the feedback instead and hold off reacting. You may discover your original, intense reaction was a defensive reflex, and the feedback wasn't so bad after all.

Take in the feedback and search for the bit of truth you can integrate. Of course, not all feedback is valuable, but the opportunity for awareness and the feelings it instigates makes it always of value. If you do feel provoked, it means there is some gem of truth, some nugget of importance inside the feedback. Use it as an indicator to explore yourself deeper.

The more you let the ego dissolve and instead allow your awareness to guide you, the quicker and more effectively you will receive and integrate the feedback. Think about it this way: a river flowing from mountain to ocean has many obstacles. It rolls over rocks and runs around trees and falls in the pools and meanders through canyons, and all this resistance creates these little feedback loops. Those feedback loops are where the speed of the water is changed or the water is redirected. These edges, which we call ecotones in ecology, are generally the most fertile and alive aspects of the river. These edges are where life thrives.

Embracing Feedback

The river embraces the feedback, integrates and uses those patterns to support life. You are no different, you are going to run into boulders and canyons and fall off waterfalls. You're going to plunge into deep pools. At times it will be scary. You may not know where you are. You won't always know where the feedback takes you, but there is one thing you can be sure of. One pattern that you can rely on. Every one of those perceived obstacles and every bit of that feedback provide fertile ground for your personal growth. Fertile ground for your life. Fertile ground for your business. Fertile ground for your relationships.

Living in this way helps you align with what is. It is nonresistance to the truth of life. Aligning what is can catalyze you to accomplish goals and reach milestones. By accepting and integrating feedback, you honor the hard truths that are around you. You honor what you don't know. You humble yourself in the face of the world and your humility creates space for natural processes to thrive. The more you accept feedback and align yourself with the truth of life, the clearer your path will become. You will know what adjustments to make and your momentum will be unstoppable.

Sowing Togetherness

What are the ways of being, the activities and processes that bring people together? As inherently tribal and social creatures, exploring these aspects of ourselves can lead to a restoration of our troubled relationships. A healing of our fractured communities. More than ever, the human community needs to find ways to bridge our separation and build bridges of peace. This task may prove the most important as actions we take can save humankind and life on the planet.

Violence, war, racism, discrimination—these are products of separation, whether on a societal level or an individual one. Implementing methods to sow togetherness is one of our greatest and most urgent tasks in the world today. As we know, attentive listening is a great tool we can use, but what are other ways we can bring people together? As social creatures there exists many modalities for human connection. Sometimes we may take the simple forms of connection for granted.

I believe the simple ways to connect may be the most effective. We can utilize seemingly everyday activities to bring us together. Sports, school, sharing food, art, work, gym, yoga, gardening, all provide good points of connection in your community. You can decide how you leverage these different forms the community takes to gather and socialize. With intention you may be able to instigate a stronger connection. Often it just takes the willingness to be open. To put a small bit of effort towards something beyond the surface connection much of the western world functions upon.

If you are bold with a mission to sow togetherness, you can start by engaging in authentic conversations with people. Share true aspects of who you are and you will be surprised what others share with you. Give the gift of listening and discover how alike your struggles and dreams are with other people. Connect authentically but remember to set healthy boundaries to protect yourself. Also respect the boundaries of others. This builds trust, ensuring the connection avoids getting polluted by negative stories and emotions. Make it your mission to be kind to others even if you don't agree with them. Cultivate a practice of being generous, sensitive and compassionate, and watch the bonds of togetherness weave a connected world.

The Best in People

As emotional pollinators, we know we can affect other people with our words and actions. We also know that with awareness, acceptance and love, we can pollinate joy in our relationships and in the world. One technique for accomplishing this is recognizing the good in each person. Once we can recognize this in another, we can choose to speak directly to that part of them.

I always try speaking to the best in others. I listen beyond the words, beyond the stories, and I look for the beauty in that person's soul. Every person has what I imagine to be a perfect and beautiful gem inside of them. This is where their capacity for love, happiness and dignity resides. I fundamentally believe in people's ability to be good. Through my own experiences I have seen "problem people" respond to love and kindness. People even who are considered "difficult" can show their beauty in incredible ways when the space is provided for their beauty to shine. Treat every person with respect and nurture the goodness in them. You don't have to support or agree with their ideas but you can listen without judgment, share your empathy, or support with compassion and understanding on a human-to-human level.

We have to remember for many people, the safe space or container needs to be there for them to step into. If we go through life without awareness or presence of others and we use our own ego-driven needs to fill the space everywhere we go, then we don't get to experience the beauty of others. The more we create space for others to shine in, the more connected we can become with each other. Put aside your judgments of each other. Bring the focus of relationships back to listening, reconciliation, compassion and love. Our traumatic histories have created seemingly permanent divisions between people and cultures. But these walls are held up by assumptions. They are bolstered by the repression of our truths and fears of judgment. By connecting with the best in people, we create space for healing to occur. We build new connections of love and solidarity. Let's tear down the walls that keep us apart and feed the beauty growing inside us all.

Giving love and generosity to one another must be done without an expectation of return or a specific outcome to be achieved. This unconditional giving respects your own self-worth and dignity along with the worth of others. To give with love, for the act alone, is true generosity.

Nourish your relationships with good communication, take the fifth mission ...

Mission: Communicate Your Truth
Go to Page 182

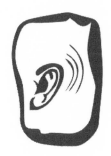

Three Levels

1. A Small Gesture of Truth
2. Develop a Support System and Reflect
3. Transformation Milestone

CHAPTER 6

LOVE IS GENEROSITY

"Compassion and tolerance are not a sign of weakness, but a sign of strength."
—Dalai Lama

Compassion and Generosity

Compassion is connection. The connection of your heart and your love for others. It is your love for all life that is shared freely. Compassion is the ability to hold space for other's pain, to accept reality and support the healing processes. This is the way of compassionate people. When you are present, deep in awareness, compassion will come unhindered. It is a natural state humans can cultivate with intention.

Often when things get tough or someone does something you deem wrong, compassion can unlock solutions and heal emotional wounds. Being compassionate allows you to stay gentle even during negative situations. You can feed a situation with love and kindness when it is needed most.

Compassion is a state of being while generosity is compassion in action. Generosity is the unifying glue keeping our humanity intact. The more we show up for each other, support and care for one another, the better quality of life all people will have. People who are treated kindly and with respect will often pass that gift on to others naturally. Being generous is like planting a little seed of love in someone to sprout and take root.

The trick to living a generous life is to make sure you don't expect anything in return. To give to someone with expectations of them, be it time or material possession, can become a dangerous and manipulative form of control over that person. Likely, you will set yourself up for disappointment, causing more suffering when the person you helped doesn't meet your expectations. In many cases, we don't communicate our expectations in the first place. We expect so much, we think others will read our minds or sense what we want from them in return for our generosity. They don't even know we have expectations. They will never fulfill our unspoken wants but for some crazy reason we expect this anyway!

If you need a return for being generous, there is a grand prize you receive if you're humble enough. Something more useful and potent than anything another person can give you. It is the joy you feel for sharing your love through generosity. The feeling of unconditionally caring for others. Bringing peace and nurturing to their lives. This is the greatest bestowal you can receive from your generosity. Generosity can fill your whole life with joy. This love leaves a powerful mark in the community. The more you give in this way, the deeper joy grows in your heart. You tap into the eternal well of love that is the universe. The more you access this well, the happier your life and the life of those around you become.

The Great Garden Giveaway

We are all powerful agents for generating love in our communities. Activating this aspect of ourselves can have lasting effects for ourselves and the world we live in. I began my journey in my teenage years, setting the trajectory of my adult life ...

From 1998–1999, I took major first steps onto this lifelong path. After experiencing an opportunity to engage in the Headwaters Forest Initiative of Humboldt County, California, an effort to protect the last stands of old-growth redwoods, I became inspired to commit myself to doing work to better the planet.

I was living in a converted garage at the time, with my two best friends who happened to be brothers. I didn't feel comfortable in my home because of what was happening with my mom, so the age of eighteen I moved in with my friends. Energized by a sense of freedom and the world at my fingertips, I began a path of fierce independence.

One of my friends (the older of the two brothers), was in a college program where students had to choose a real project to use as their thesis. One night we stayed up late talking about what his project would be. He and some other classmates were talking about various possibilities. The ultimate goal to do something positive for the community and the Earth. Emerging from these vision sessions was a project rooted in generosity to tend the community and environment in the region where we lived. We called it the Great Garden Giveaway. The plan was to give gardens away to the community using special heirloom and traditional seed types (seventy-five-year-old varieties and older). Our goal was to connect people with the land and their food, while at the same time growing and preserving these old and rare seed varieties as a means of protecting biodiversity and generating food security.

Planting Earth Activation

Several months later, we turned this glorious dream into a reality. We started a nonprofit organization we called Planting Earth Activation. We called it P.E.A. There we were, a group of young idealistic youth in our late teens to early twenties, devoting ourselves to changing the world with generosity. We were not only driven by our mission of doing good but also by grief, anger, and fear of the large-scale, corporate privatization of basic life needs like water, seeds, food, and energy. At the same time, we were still hopeful and optimistic; we wanted to do something that would benefit everyone and all people could get behind regardless of race, gender, class, religion or politic ideology. The garden seemed like the perfect place to weave these goals together.

It was a powerful notion then and it's still a powerful vision of what's possible. Everyone on this planet eats food. I believe everyone on this planet deserves and has the right to access, grow and consume healthy food. Passionate and idealistic, we set out to transform ourselves and our community. We were determined for this to succeed. We elicited donations from friends and family to get us going. We were able to get donated materials like compost, planting pots, seeds, and tools. We secured a place at the local community garden to launch our new Garden Giveaway campaign. We organized a large volunteer garden party to kick off the project. It was an epic launch. It felt like a movement.

This was an amazing time in my life and in the city where I lived. We launched a new garden party every few months, spending the in-between time organizing new garden projects, materials, volunteers, and promotion. Our main target for garden projects were people's front yard lawns. Neighborhood by neighborhood, we knocked on the doors of lawn owners to offer them a free garden. Our goals were to work neighborhood by neighborhood so we could complete multiple gardens on the same garden festival day. We called these "neighborhood food webs," as our grand plan was for neighbors to grow what was optimal in their microclimate, topography and sun orientation. The final goal was to have neighbors trade and share food with each other.

Could you imagine how this would all go down? A stranger knocks on your door. You open the door to a young activist. This young person proceeds to offer to turn your lawn into a garden, completely free! Folks would often look perplexed by the prospect of receiving a free garden. In most cases people responded positively, proceeding to receive a free garden from us. Below is a first-hand account of one our first planting festivals and the awesome power of generosity...

The High Street Planting Party

The High Street Planting Party was one of our first and biggest planting festivals. I woke up that first morning feeling inspired and excited. The mission we were embarking on seemed unprecedented at the time and it gave me the chills. I was about to spend the whole day working outside with my community, building gardens and growing food together. What could be better?

This festival was composed of eight gardens spread across two city blocks. Most of them were front yards along with a few backyards. We had a leader and support person for every garden. We were highly organized; we had garnered the support of sixty-plus volunteers for the day. We had twenty yards of compost delivered. We had support from the innovative city we were operating in, along with the required signatures of residents to officially shut down the block to car traffic. We built a stage in the street and had musicians, dancers and artists performing on stage and roving from garden to garden while volunteers worked to prep and plant.

Not only were we building front yard community gardens, but we were connecting neighbor to neighbor, and neighborhood to neighborhood. People of all walks of life, culture, religion, race, and class came together in these gardens.

My days with Planting Earth Activation set me clearly on the path I've been navigating the last twenty years. It's through the development of this organization and those experiences, that I deepened my relationship with the planet and its diverse cultures, and strengthened my resolve to tend to nature and community. The generosity, love and action we took gave rise to a series of endeavors, businesses, campaigns and projects nourishing our community and ourselves. Little did I know at the time, but I was also gaining vital skills I would need to thrive in my life and career.

Your Most Essential Project

You are you most essential project. Everything you want to accomplish in the world. All the vision you have for your life. The quality of your relationships all have one thing in common. You.

Get clear about what really matters to you. Peel back the layers of programming about who you think you should be. Connect with your passions and know your stressors. When you get to the core of who are, you will realize just how much you need your own attention. Rather than placing all of your worth in the judgment of others or temporary material gain, you find acceptance and love from within. If you make health and happiness the biggest priority in your life, you will find it easier to spread positive energy to others.

Giving yourself the love you need doesn't mean that you ignore the world. Your world can actually grow bigger as you are drawn to what makes you happy. The effort you put forth will be energized and more effective when rooted in your own life purpose. Give yourself the nourishment you need. Become your own master healer. Become your own master life coach, and empower a joyful life. Little by little, day by day, slow and steady practice yields the best results. Reprogramming is a muscle that has to be exercised. Read this book ten times if you have too!

The Generosity of Heart-Centered Leadership

In this world, on a large scale, we see too few leaders who lead with the generosity of the heart. We see many who lead by force, coercion, manipulation and fanatical egos. While love-based leadership is scarce, there are some notable examples, like the Dalai Lama. By leading with the heart, we create an atmosphere of peace and a space for truthful communication and reconciliation. Whether it is community or small business scale or at an institutional level, this approach further provides the potential to support cultures of forgiveness and healing.

These qualities and actions in our leadership, organizations and businesses create long-lasting, thriving models of collective organizing. It also puts our own needs at the center of everything we do, as leading from the heart begins with self-love. As a result, this type of leadership generates beautiful community interactions, making way for miraculous things to happen. I believe everyone has some kind of intrinsic leadership skills inside of them. With leadership, our task is to motivate, inspire, support or organize with others. Much of our culture recognizes intellectual leadership as the most revered. While it is hugely important to understand the scientific facts of the system that a leader is organizing, it is not the only trait needed to be an effective leader. Many of the most effective and passionate leaders don't lead only from their mind, but from their heart as well. They still acknowledge the important use of knowledge and science, but not as the sole frame for making decisions and taking action.

Authentic leadership comes from the heart. And it's a powerful tool in the regeneration of our communities and planet. To lead with the heart is to be humble, to know what you don't know, to deeply listen to those you work with or influence. Those that lead with the heart, that use compassion, empathy, and understanding as a way to build bridges and provide sound leadership, provide a great service to the world.

Someone who leads in this way activates the leadership and empowerment of those around them. Someone who leads with the heart is not always driven by ego, prestige, or power. They lead by being who they are. They lead by being true to themselves. It is a brave act to be true to yourself. This courage comes in the form of authentic communication and positive action. Once released, generosity and compassion spreads and grows everywhere.

To spread kindness everywhere, take the sixth mission ...

Mission: Actions of Generosity
Go to Page 185

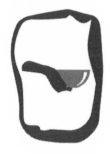

Three Levels

1. A Kind Deed
2. Actions of Generosity
3. Be a Peacemaker

PART THREE:
TRANSFORMATION

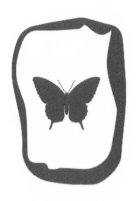

To heal the wounds of your heart,
Forgive all those that hurt you so,
Forgive the grief that you hold,
Forgive all you can't control.

CHAPTER 7
SEEDS OF GRIEF

"These pains you feel are messengers.
Listen to them."
—Rumi

The Wall of Grief

Already, you have stepped into an awakening journey to activate the joy of who you are. By now, reading this book, you may see yourself and the world with new eyes. By completing some or all of the missions up to this point, you have bravely taken responsibility for your own happiness and your vision for your life. But something else may have happened during this process. You may have found yourself running into obstacles that trip you up during your missions and reflections. You may have run into an emotional wall. A wall of grief. A wall of doubt. A wall of fear.

The incredible and courageous work of transforming your stories and dissolving your ego extracts the strongest and most traumatic beliefs in your mind. These long-held frames of thinking, these limiting beliefs, may stem from potent events that happened to you in your life. You may not even remember them. This grief may also come from generations of trauma, pain and programmed thinking passed to you by your parents, grandparents and ancestors. You get to choose what you do with this grief. Keep it locked away? Accept and heal? Face your deepest fears? Implementing the missions in this book can bring up a lot. They can shed light on what is true and what is not. It can seem like your whole world is not what you thought it was. There may be fear of making these large-scale changes in your life, your relationships, and your work. You might feel potential outcomes are too mysterious, too risky. The fear and doubt that ripples on the surface of your mind, this is just another story of the mind. An illusion, yes, but one that can feel insurmountably powerful.

Moments of Opportunity

We don't want to ignore the big walls of grief that show up in this process. These are moments of great opportunity. The missions related to this part of the book are going to be change-makers for you. Seeds to launch your new, limitless way of living and mark important milestones toward fully accepting yourself and others. The secret to transforming these foundational beliefs starts with acknowledging them. Recognition means allowing yourself to feel and accept the emotions that surface. Feel them fully. From there you can find the power to forgive.

Recognizing the seeds of our grief is a sacred and courageous practice. In western cultures, we are not taught how to navigate the water of grief. We are more often than not, taught to suppress. Taught to forget, taught to master with force, rather than acknowledge with our vulnerable truths.

Stay the course that unveils itself while you work through your transformation processes. Grief will arise. Fear will try to build a wall between you and your awakened purpose. Most of all, doubt will creep in to the spaces of your mind, telling you you're not good enough. These are tests. They are rites of passage that every one of us must work through to live in truth and self-love.

What has been frightening for me in my own process is when I opened myself up to the truths of the world we live in. Once I began to learn the truths of the violent and terrible parts of our world, I knew there was an unfathomable amount of healing to be done. Healing in myself, my family, my community and throughout humanity. My awakening left me feeling overwhelmed by the work I felt needed to be done. The work to making peace. The work to steward and restore our ecosystems. The work of living in harmony with each other and the planet.

Sometimes it seems insurmountable, almost silly to think that you have any part to play. But you do have a part to play. That's why the seeds of grief arise in you. You are the result of everything that happened before. The trials of your ancestors. The evolution of the planet. The results of the choices you've made in your life. And we often stumble into this connection to the past. The stories (often generational) control our frames, our cultural identity and how we think we're supposed to be in the world. Often the image you project of who you are to the world, is deeply informed by the stories of the past. As you question those stories and work to align with the truth of who are in the world you will eventually slam into that wall of grief.

A Message from the Ancestors

In my early twenties I found myself in this exact situation. Since I was eighteen, I had devoted myself to activism and learning about how to restore the planet. My journey to this point was fraught with doubt and fear. For the most part I felt my family's concern at me ditching college to start a nonprofit community gardening organization and pursue my activist aspirations. I felt dedicated to my work and clearly on my path but without the support of my family or society, I also felt on the fringe. I didn't actually know how I would support myself doing my activism. I wasn't really sure what I was doing other than following my heart and passions. Overtime, the seeds of grief welled up in me to an almost breaking point. Then something amazing happened to me. The following is the story of one of the most powerful dreams I have ever had. This dream helped me break through my own wall of grief and embrace the life path I had stepped onto.

It was a foggy summer day, and my friend and I had taken the weekend to go on a backpacking trip in the Point Reyes National Seashore. That first day was a wonderful hike through a resurgent coastal-forest ecosystem. This particular land had experienced a forest fire about a decade prior and I remember the miracle of seeing so much life and abundant growth of the forest in those ten years since the fire.

Our campsite for the night was directly on the beach alongside Drakes Bay and the Pacific Ocean. Rather than sleeping in a tent we decided to sleep right on the beach underneath the night sky. It had been a lovely day and I enjoyed laying my head to rest looking up at the stars above. I fell into a deep sleep and soon found myself in the middle of a profound dream.

Dreaming of My Abuelo

I was standing at the edge of a sparkling swimming pool filled with water. I looked around and saw an outdoor table and chairs meant for hanging out around the pool. All of a sudden I heard a voice. I recognized that voice. That's the voice of my Abuelo. My Abuelo was my mother's grandfather, my great-grandfather. He grew up in Argentina and never spoke a word of English. It was strange to be understanding his words now for I never fully learned how to speak Spanish as a child and he and I were never able to communicate effectively with our words.

While we didn't speak each other's languages we were still very close throughout my childhood. He was a funny, friendly and animated man with great love in his heart. When I was thirteen years old my Abuelo passed away. It was one of the first great losses I'd ever experienced. After he had passed away, his daughter, my Abuelita (grandmother), had given me a special medal that my Abuelo had won in Argentina during a bike race. I wore this medal around my neck daily as a reminder of him. It was my talisman and sacred to me. I was wearing it this night as I fell asleep on the beach.

My Abuelo was talking to me and I could understand what he was saying. I sat down at the table to have a conversation with him. It was so wonderful to see him there. He told me he had an important message for me. He told me that he had been watching me and knew of all of the work I have been doing in the world. He told me he could feel the fears and doubts surrounding me and this path I had chosen. I sat and listened, feeling slightly shocked and in awe at what he was saying. He told me it was okay. He said it was okay to feel all the things I was feeling and not to worry.

Then he told me something with a strong conviction: "Erik, you are on the right path now. Do not doubt what you are doing. Do not worry about what others think you should or should not be doing. You are needed in this time and I want you to know that everything is going to work out, okay? Erik, the path you are on is not going to be easy. There are great challenges ahead of you, but I need you to know, do not give up. Stay committed to your mission and to yourself. Stay connected to the Earth and everything will be okay. I believe in you Erik and I'm here for you."

I thanked my Abuelo, giving him a huge hug and the customary Argentine kisses on his cheek. He smiled at me as my dream faded away and I woke up. It was the middle of the night and the sliver of a moon hung amongst the stars. My friend was sleeping next to me. I crawled out of my sleeping bag and knelt onto the sand. I rested my forehead on the ground and began crying deeply. My fears and my doubts washing away into the sand. I was breaking through the wall of grief.

In that moment, I made a vow to myself and to the Earth. I vowed to stay on the path I had chosen no matter what trials awaited me. I shared my gratitude for my ancestors and for my life. I knelt there crying and praying for at least forty-five minutes before I crawled back to my sleeping bag and fell asleep again for the night.

Accepting My Path

This was a powerful moment for me as I fully accepted the trajectory of my life and felt the support of my ancestors. This would not be the last time I had to face my fears. My Abuelo has never come back to me in a dream although I feel his presence when I write these words. I didn't realize it at the time but my dream also helped me process the grief I still held from his death.

The next years of my life I would launch into a myriad of passion projects and campaigns. All of them brought up the same fears and griefs as before, but this time I had faith in myself. This time I knew what these walls were about. The seeds of grief that stem from living in truth are constant reminders to me of how important it is to be a peace maker in the world and how that peace only comes from the vitality of my own self-love.

How would I know that even greater challenges would test that resolve? How would I know the greatest tests were yet to come and they would change me forever? Just when I thought I could navigate my grief, the greatest loss of my life turned my world upside down. When you're ready, read the next chapter to find out what happened ...

CHAPTER 8

DEATH TRANSFORMING LIFE

"There is sacredness in tears. They are not the mark of weakness, but of power. They speak more eloquently than ten thousand tongues. They are the messengers of overwhelming grief, of deep contrition, and of unspeakable love."
—Washington Irving

A Day of Unraveling

Throughout our lives there are certain events and experiences that mark major shifts in who we are and how we see the world. These moments of change, growth and potential unraveling become a turning point in our journey through life. The following story is a day like this for me.

August 1, 2008

The day started out like any other day. There were a handful of appointments and tasks to be done, which kicked off with a visit to one of my landscaping projects. I was meeting my dad at the job site and loading up a tractor for transport. My wife and our six-month child, had gone to a mom and baby group for new mothers. Later that day, my wife, son and I met up and headed together to the pediatrician's office. Time for a well check up on our baby boy. My wife reported how our son had been having a tough day. He had been crying and colicky, making it difficult to be at the mothers group.

Six long months as new parents were taking their toll on us. Our little guy wasn't a great sleeper and we were not great non-sleepers. It had been pretty intense lately and we were all sleep deprived. Going to the pediatrician was never a fun experience as our boy did not like being weighed or measured on top of anything else! The appointment lasted about an hour, going as well as can be expected. Our son's weight was on track, he was healthy and growing strong. Getting in the car to drive home, my phone rang. A phone call that changed my life forever. I will never forget this moment, the words that were spoken and the powerful emotions that erupted inside me.

First, let's back up one day before this phone call ...

July 31, 2008

My mother was moving on this day. She was leaving a condo her soon to be ex-husband had relocated her too when they had separated and sold the house they had owned together. She was moving across town to a new, more comfortable home of her own. This was a big rite of passage for her. She was at the end of a nasty divorce and this new living situation removed the last ties to her soon-to-be ex-husband.

While this was a milestone achieved, my mother had still fallen prey to her own depression and the move seemed anticlimactic for her. Dark stories emerged out of the large changes happening in her life. My siblings and I joined together to help make this a smooth transition to her new dwelling. Not only did she need the physical brawn to move her stuff, but the emotional support as well. My siblings and I were all pretty new parents at this time, with young children and babies. It was always a great time when we all got together with our mother. We all enjoyed seeing our children getting to play with their Nonna. Nonna and her grandchildren got to hang out while we moved my mom's stuff into her new house.

It was a long day of loading up trucks, moving her stuff across town, unloading, and making sure Mom and the kids had what they needed as evening approached. We did our best to get her house set up for her first night staying there. It was a long day but it felt great to see my mom in her new place. Was a new chapter finally beginning for her? A life with less pain and stress? Maybe she would pick up a new hobby or meet some new friends in this new community. I was optimistic.

That night, while getting ready for bed, I received a phone call from my mother. Through the answering machine, I could hear her saying she was looking for a remote control for the TV. She had been searching in boxes everywhere and couldn't find it. It was late at night, we were trying to get our baby boy down to sleep, and I didn't pick up the phone nor call her back. I didn't know where the remote control was anyway.

I remember feeling proud of my mother for making this big shift and moving into her new house, feeling hopeful about how our family had unified behind her. That day, my siblings and I and our children were brought together by our love for our mother. It was time for my mom to feel independent again. Time for her to take control of her life, and heal from her past traumas ...

The next day ... August 1 2008

As I pulled away from the pediatrician's office the phone rang. I pick up the call. My sister's voice sounded shaky. She had big news but was having a hard time telling me.

"A terrible accident and ... and ..." she stuttered.

With my heart fluttering, I said, "What is it? What happened? Just tell me."

My sister, still hesitating, said, "Where are you, what are you doing?"

Anxiety growing, I told her, "I'm pulling away from the doctor's office, please tell me what's going on."

"Okay, okay." She whispered. I heard the franticness in her voice. "Erik, Mom is dead." My world started spinning. "There was an accident and she's dead, she's dead."

Like a tsunami striking the shore, my whole body shuttered. "What! What, what happened?"

"We are at her house, we don't know what happened, can you come here right now?" She asked. My wife and son picked up on the intensity of the moment, as tears streamed down my face.

I told my wife. "We need to drive to my mom's house right now can you drive? She's dead, my momma's dead." Another tremor moved through my body as a primal emotional release took over.

I can't believe it. I can't believe it. Oh my God, I was just with her yesterday. She only had one night in her new home. This can't be real. Is this real? I thought to myself.

We rushed to Mom's house, twenty minutes away. My brave wife was trying to drive calmly while supporting me and our little boy. He was picking up on the emotional crisis and had started to cry as well. We arrived. My two sisters, brother and brother-in-law were already there, along with police officers. We all stood there in shock.

Discovering Loss

My sister hadn't heard from my mom all that morning and after calling numerous times, decided to head over to make sure she was okay. When she and her husband arrived, they found the doors locked. My mother wasn't responding to knocking or the doorbell ringing. My sister and brother-in-law tried to find a way into the house, checking windows and doors. In growing desperation, my brother-in-law grabbed a ladder to a second floor window. My sister, sensing something was wrong, decided she needed to be the one to go in first. There was one window which she had left unlocked the night before. She pushed it open and crawled inside the house ...

She searched the house, unable to find our mom in her bedroom. She went down to the garage. My mother was sitting on a step, slumped forward. Quiet, asleep, dead. She screamed for my brother-in-law and ran to let him in the house. I can't imagine what this must have been like for my sister. She asked her husband to check our mom's vital signs not wanting to do it herself. He confirmed our mother's passing, then covered our deceased mother with a blanket.

The Choice I Made

The big question remained. How did our mother pass away sitting there on the steps? It didn't make sense and with trepidation, we knew there was more to the story. I walked into my mother's house knowing her body was still in the garage. My sister told me I could go see my mother's body if I wanted to. I was terrified and stood paralyzed. I didn't want my last image of my mother being her dead body. Fear gripped me thoroughly as grief and shock settled in. I chose not to see her. To this day I still regret that decision.

I wish I had the courage to see her once more. To hold her hand, to whisper to her. Tell her everything was okay. To tell her the pain is over. You don't have to fear anymore, Momma. You are loved, you are worthy. I wanted to say these things to her, but she was gone. What was I supposed do now? How could I tell her I wished for more time with her? That I was not ready for her to leave. My baby boy was only six months. He needed his Nona ... I needed my mother ...

How could I tell her all the blame I feel? How could I tell her I wish I was courageous enough to help her more? I knew how much she was hurting. I knew it was only matter of time before something like this happened. We all did. Not because we thought she would take her own life. The love she felt for her children and grandchildren was too compelling. No matter how much pain she was in, I don't think she would ever abandon us intentionally ...

Only She Could Save Herself

But her pain, her trauma, the stories she had about herself, the stories she held about others were powerful illusions she had invested her life energy into. She could never figure out how to let them go. She kept hitting her wall of grief, unable to transform it. Unable to acknowledge the truth behind her pain and surrender to it.

People with this level of depression often look for escapes. We knew she had been addicted to painkillers. In the heart-wrenching last ten years of her life, she had gone in and out of health emergencies. Sadly, she ended up hooked on prescription drugs and the emotional roller coaster that went with it. On the day before she died, she had promised that she had stopped using those drugs. My sister had confronted her about this when Mom walked in the house with a bag from the pharmacy. "I've been off opiates for months," Mom had said.

The Truth of What Happened

Later, on the day we found her body, we were organizing my mother's possessions and found two empty bottles of a powerful, injectable opiate. Her doctor had given it to her the same day we helped her move into her new house. There was no reason for this doctor to give her this medicine. My mom, being a nurse, gave herself the injections based on her doctor's recommendation. A few weeks later, the coroner's report revealed what we already suspected. Her cause of death: an overdose on a prescription drug seven times more powerful than morphine.

Cycles of Life and Death

The day my mother passed away was a day of unraveling. A day to face my greatest and darkest fears. A day to test the resilience of myself. After we had finished up at my mom's house, we went to my sister's house to have dinner, recuperate and process what happened. Once we got there, I felt an intense need to be by myself. I needed to connect with nature in some way so I stepped out into my sister's backyard. There was a large beautiful live oak there and I found a place to sit on the ground and feel what was building inside my body.

I collapsed onto the ground, as wave after wave of grief-stricken emotion poured through me. It was a full body, deeply soulful experience. I let myself go completely as it turned into loud, uncontrollable howling. My family became worried, and came to the back door to make sure I was okay. I let them know I was fine but I still needed to have my process. This went on for a good hour. Finally, a calm surfaced inside me. I found myself face down on the ground. I had scratched out a dent for my body in the layers of thick mulch and oak leaves.

Revelation

I came to the present moment and was able to see the oak tree for what it was. A sentinel of life. A life-giving home for owls and squirrels. A gift to humans and all living things by the oxygen it exhales and carbon it sequesters. I felt such gratitude for its beauty. I found myself holding its yellow, cracked and decaying leaves. Digging in the mulch with my hands,

I found acorns sprouting. I dug deeper into dark, woody material until I reached soil. Fungi, worms, sow bugs, the ground was teaming with life. Beneath the layers of dead and decaying leaves, the blessing and birth of life was commencing.

Life, death, and birth. A cycle of regeneration. The grand cycle of nature. Life, born from the gift left by past generations. Surrendering to the grief of losing of my mother opened me to what I felt was a greater understanding of the universe. I experienced a moment of unbelievable clarity. A precious moment of awareness, a connection with the oneness of all life. I began to feel better, and with a deep sigh of release I sent a prayer to my mother. A prayer of gratitude for all she taught and sacrificed for me. A prayer for her safe travels, for her freedom and for her peace.

Healing Love

I stood up, going inside to hold my six-month-old son. It had been an intense emotional day for him too, and I hadn't given him the kind of attention I wanted too. I held him in my arms and I looked into his eyes. Looking into his eyes, I noticed a miracle. I saw my mother looking back at me … My son had her eyes … Then my lesson with the oak tree rooted deeper. My mother's legacy, the gift of life she gave me, enabled me to give life too, the life of my baby boy …

The love of my son and wife was the greatest support system I could have received during the grief-laden months following my mom's passing. One generation moved on, yet a new generation had just arrived. My child, so innocent and open, ready to experience the magic of the world. I poured my heart into that little guy. I vowed to teach him the best of what my mom had taught me. She was a principled and passionate philosopher, activist and historian. A lover of people and nature. A healer and an inspiration. She was braver in her freedom of expression beyond anyone I have ever met.

I'm filled with gratitude at what she taught me about the world. She imparted a social framework of the world, educating me about the need for equality, justice, and peace. She cultivated in me an appreciation and wonderment of the natural world and compassion for all living things.

Most of all, my mother demonstrated how to love strong and love fiercely. To care for others and the world with fiery passion is her legacy. These are the seeds that she has planted in the world. The seeds that have sprouted inside me and carry on in the life of my daughter and my son. Like the leaves that turn to soil, feeding the sprouting acorn, these are the cycles of life and death and the birth of a new generation.

If you are ready for transformation, take the seventh mission ...

Mission: Face Your Grief
Go to Page 188

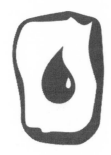

Four Levels

1. Heal a grievance
2. The Grief Altar
3. Create Grief Ritual
4. Make an Agreement

CHAPTER 9
THE HEALING POWER FORGIVENESS

"Forgiveness is the only way to heal your emotional wounds.
Forgive those who hurt you no matter what they've done
because
you don't want to hurt yourself every time you remember what
they did.
When you can touch a wound and it doesn't hurt,
then you know you have truly forgiven."
—Don Miguel Ruiz

The Letter of Forgiveness

The fear of forgiving another person unearths complex and confusing emotions. Both the self-judgment and the judgment of others become obstacles to cope with. See through the fear. An act of forgiveness is an act of healing. Possibly the most instrumental healing to be activated in humanity.

A wise man once told me, "To forgive another person, one must forgive themselves first." Both must to be forgiven. Forgive yourself first and your act to forgive another will be true. Forgive myself first? How do I even do that? What if I'm not sure what I'm supposed to be forgiving myself for? These are tough questions and the answers are found throughout this entire book. To forgive another person takes courage. For me, it brings up all my fear of conflict, which usually leads me to anxiety. The following story captures a personal experience where I found the courage to forgive despite my fear.

In my early twenties, a mentor of mine sponsored me to take a special personal development forum. I went to the opening talk to see what it was like prior to deciding on the program. It was a surreal experience. There was a lot of flair and energy about the people that presented. This was startlingly authentic to me. So much so, I actually felt uncomfortable at times. I was intrigued enough and decided to take the three-day seminar.

I made the right decision. The program turned out to be a life-changing experience for me. What I learned became foundational to living a life true to myself. The big Aha moment came on the last day. The day before, an assignment was given to write a letter to someone who you wanted to clear the air with. Someone you wanted to forgive or ask for forgiveness from. I chose to write a letter to my dad. Ever since my parents divorced, my relationship with my dad had become more and more strained. Particularly the tension came from stories I had made up about him. Stories I believed with a self-sabotaging intensity.

Believing My Illusions (Back Story) …

I was nineteen or twenty years old. I hadn't gone to college yet and I was considering attending the local college where my dad worked. My dad offered to support me financially so I could start taking classes. It was a generous offer and I took the chance. His agreement had one stipulation. If I dropped out, I would have to pay him the money back. I've never been competent in classroom environments and after a few months, I dropped out of most classes. At the same time in my life, I had stepped onto my path in permaculture and land restoration work. Going to college had actually become an obstacle to me taking off as a young ecological designer and community organizer.

I didn't have much money in this era of life, and of course, I couldn't pay my dad back once I dropped out. I kept the facts hidden from him as long as I could because I was scared of his judgment. Eventually he discovered that I had dropped out of school. I knew—or thought I knew—he was extremely disappointed with me. I enabled myself to make up stories about what he was thinking. I told myself he thought I was lazy, a slack off, lost, out of integrity.

Consumed by dread, I never chose the direct route of talking to him about it. I ignorantly believed my own story. I sabotaged my relationship with my dad in this way. I never gave him the chance for our truths to be told. Not my truth, nor his truth. I avoided talking with him about this in any way I could. This did not lead to bridging the gaps in our relationship.

Looking back, I can see I was damaging many of my familial relationships. Since my family was mostly college-educated professionals, I thought they wouldn't consider me worthy if I didn't go to college. The work in landscape design and activism was the right path for me, but I kept feeling that no one else believed in me. My mother, the notable exception, was the only one actively supporting my emerging destiny. With everyone else, I felt a large disconnection. I had found a new sort of family in the friends and colleagues I was working with. I knew this community believed in me.

It turns out you can't run away forever. In the end, we always have to face ourselves. We are the carrier of our own illusions. My resentment of my dad and all the ways I wish he would support me became a heavy burden to carry. I had let these fears fester, which led to depression, low self-esteem, and a sacrificial frame of mind. In truth, my pain was rooted in the deep love I carried for him and the disappointment of what felt like an unhealthy relationship. Always craving joy in my relationship with him. Always wanting to share my passions with him and hear his point of view with compassion. This is what I truly yearned for.

Back at the program ...

I chose to write a letter to my dad that second day at the seminar I was attending. It was time to share my truth with him. Time to apologize for my shortcomings, for my lies, for my distance. Writing the letter was a great first step to forgiving myself and my dad. I wasn't sure I would actually send the letter to him but for my own healing process, writing the letter was a breakthrough. I didn't know that was only the beginning.

My letter in hand, I started the last day of the program. The facilitator looked for acknowledgment that participants had written their letters. "Now the next step is upon us," she stated. The task of this day was to call the subject of your letter and read it to them. What?! I thought, feeling anxious energy course through my body as my stomach dropped. I was terrified.

Thoughts of escape immediately surfaced. *There is no way I'm going to call. I'm not putting myself in that situation. There are over one hundred people in this room, no one will notice if I skip this exercise. They can't make me, right? Call and read this letter to my dad? Maybe, maybe I'd be okay sending it to him in the mail and I'll wait in the shadows until he reaches out to me. I mean, what if I call him and read the letter and he confirms all my deepest fears about how unworthy I am? What if he tells me how much I failed him? What a disappointment I am? What if he tells me the path I've chosen leads nowhere? I'm sure that's what he's going to say if I call him.*

Some folks in the program had the courage to go first. They walked into private side rooms to make their calls. I held out as long as I could. After a couple hours went by, something happened that changed everything. A woman emerged from her phone call with a powerful story to share. She was an older woman who endured a falling out with her dad. It had lasted nearly fifty years. Recently her dad had passed away and she held many unresolved feelings about him. The person she called was his ex-wife. It turned out this woman in my program had been living a lie. I don't remember the details of her story but she had been told a story of actions her dad had taken, and completely stopped talking to him for all those years. She had spoken to her father's ex-wife, and found that the story she heard was wrong.

Right in front of my eyes I saw her whole world flip around. She began sharing the many decisions she'd made in her life because of the stories about her dad. This discovery led to a lot of regret that she processed right in the room with us. Her main emotion was relief among the shock. When she was done sharing her story she seemed younger, lighter, and more joyful.

I sat in stunned silence at the gravity of what I had just heard. Fifty years of being estranged from her father, all for a lie? Was I doing the same thing with my dad? What lies had I led myself to believe? I didn't want to wait until my dad passed away decades from now to learn and live the truth. I felt a rise of courage and resolve in my heart. It was time to call my dad and read him this letter. I got up and walked into the phone room ...

Reading the Letter

I sat down at the phone, my heart aflutter. I pulled out the two-page letter I had written my dad. The letter that exposed the story I believe about him. The letter that represented the limiting stories I believed about myself. I picked up the receiver. I had a fleeting hope he would not be home or answer the phone. I usually didn't get a hold of him when I called and maybe he would screen a call from an unknown number. Feeling both hopeful and scared he would pick up the phone, I dialed the number.

My dad picked up the phone on the second or third ring. *Oh boy this is really happening*, I thought. He seemed in a good mood and happy to hear my voice. I proceeded to tell him I was at a conference and had written him letter. I told him I was hoping to read it to him. He didn't object and agreed to let me read through the whole letter before responding (the one rule imposed by the program).

I did it. I read the whole thing. By the end my tears were flowing. I confessed my love for him and my desire to build a good relationship. I apologized for what I felt were my shortcomings. I owned up to my lies. When I was done speaking, I braced for his reaction thinking, *here comes the hammer.*

I Was Wrong

His response was of gratitude, not judgment. I wasn't expecting that! He proceeded to share his thoughts from listening to the letter. His truth blew me away. He didn't think of me in the ways I thought he did. He apologized for his role in the distance that had grown between us. He reflected on his own escapism in not initiating this conversation himself. He took advantage of this opening to dispel the stories he believed about my feelings. His illusions were similar to mine: he feared my judgment and his perceived failing as a parent. What a crazy matrix of misperceptions and tainted beliefs we carried about each other. When he was done the air was cleared and I felt at peace.

Forgiveness is a foundation of deep healing. The body responds and feels lighter as the heart opens. Since this day I have written numerous forgiveness letters and initiated conversations like these. I find it is always difficult battling the illusions my mind makes of conflict with others. The grip of fear may be strong but the truth—my truth, your truth—will always be stronger. Forgiveness is unfailingly worth every last effort.

So, here is a question for you to ponder. Are you ready to be free? Are you ready to let go of your self-deception? Who in your life do you believe stories about? There is no need to waste another day, let alone fifty years. Do you want the truth? If you've completed the missions related to the earlier chapter in this book, then you already have the tools you need to be successful in the next mission. The *Offer of Forgiveness Mission* related to this chapter will guide you through the whole process. The moment is here. It's time to take action. Forgive yourself for being afraid. Forgive yourself for waiting so long. Express your truth and be free.

Attachment Is Pain

Attachment is a counterproductive emotion of the mind and body. When we attach ourselves to a specific outcome, a specific need or feeling we want to have, we give it a bit of our spirit. This stems from a belief that we need this attachment. The story is so compelling we often don't realize the illusory nature of the perceived need. If your attachment is strong enough, you may even feel you can't live without it or your life will lack fulfillment.

Attachments cause much pain and suffering in the world. Attachment to relationships, property ownership, material possession, money, power, these attachments lead people to hatred, violence and unspeakable acts. These are extreme outcomes but the root of these patterns rests in the basic make up of how people think and act. In some ways this is our greatest challenge to cultivating our own happiness.

We can track the arrival of attachment thinking at a young age. Parenting young children provides ample opportunity to see how these patterns play out among our most innocent. The simple act of trying to share a toy—in my house we have seen it over and over again. The challenge of building with Legos or blocks together descends into a screaming fit.

In these moments, not only are my children's attachment issues surfacing but my own as well. I'm so attached to having calm energy in the house, that when my kids start fighting and I'm out of touch with my own sense of peace, I might get angry, adding to the issue by yelling at my kids to stop fighting. Upon reflection, I find it silly that my attachment to NOT having my kids argue leads me to matching their energy with anger. This is the pure ridiculousness of attachment thinking.

The Antidote to Attachment

Acceptance and surrender are the antidote to the dark thoughts of attachment. Make acceptance a daily practice and discover how happy your life will become. If you find it difficult to jumpstart a practice, start trying to let go of small attachments.

Remember to stay in deep awareness so you can identify when you bump against small attachments. Look for those moments throughout the day. Maybe something doesn't quite go your way. For instance, you're out to eat and the food doesn't meet your satisfaction. You were late to an appointment and felt stressed and rushed getting there. In both cases, by the time the food came or you were late, there was likely nothing you could do about the situation. Yet, you may spend a ridiculous amount of time stressing about it during and after.

Maybe you were waiting for a phone call that never came or you didn't get the job you wanted. Would these normally trigger you into negative reaction? Will your attachment and all the stories that come with it turn to emotions of fear, judgment and victimhood? You can fester, feel anxious and upset, or you can surrender. The surrendering takes some of the charge out of the emotions. In this state of acceptance, you have the mental space to see other options or solutions that were unavailable when you were upset.

When I lost my ability to have normal body functions through my nervous system disorder, I experienced pain from the attachment to my old life. In fact, this has continued to represent a major test to my ability to accept my situation without attachments. Every now and then I go back through a cycle of resenting my body. Resentment that I'm not able to go more than an hour without using a bathroom and the lifestyle that accompanies it. How does this attachment to wanting to be different turn out for me? Does it help? Does it lesson the symptoms or discomfort? No it doesn't. I work on letting go of the attachment to feeling "normal." Letting go of the need to have my old life back, and that leads to epiphanies. That leads to gratitude for the beautiful life I have, and all the abundance and joy that goes with it.

With the mental and emotional capacity to make the best of a situation, you might be pleasantly surprised at the outcome. Something even better may happen due to your adjusted frame of mind. In this way, you unlock the potential of each moment.

Experience the peace that comes with forgiveness.
Take the eighth mission ...

Mission: The Gift of Forgiveness
Go to Page 192

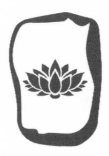

Three Levels

1. A Small Letting Go
2. The Forgiveness Letter
3. The Forgiveness Conversation

CHAPTER 10
HEALING PATHWAYS OF GRATITUDE

"In the struggle lies the joy."
—Maya Angelou

The Death of Crisis

When I was twenty-five years old, I began having intense physical symptoms. My nervous system was a wreck and I lost the functional working of my bladder. The more stressed I was, the worse the symptoms became. This triggered a vicious and seemingly endless cycle of anxiety and discomfort. Navigating these scary patterns activated the awakening of my true spirit. The whole journey of healing led me to this moment, to the words on these pages and missions of this book. At the time of writing this book, I haven't solved the chronic issue in my body, but I consider the advent of this life challenge the greatest guide to finding my joy and success in life and career.

A year and a half is how long it took me to be diagnosed after the initial symptoms began. The symptoms were so debilitating, I was unable to work or travel.

This was a very challenging, dark, and scary time for me. I forgot how to use my body in a normal way and it petrified me. Whenever you are faced with a chronic illness and especially without knowing the problem, a spiritual crisis is bound to ensue. In desperation you look for anything and everything to point the way towards diagnosing the problem. For myself, I tried everything! Western medicine, acupuncture, physical therapy, herbalism—you name it, I tried it. After seeing four different doctors, a urologist and all sorts of healers, I still made no noticeable recovery.

Searching for Answers

Distressed and exhausted, I decided to look to spiritual and emotional solutions to my situation. This led me down some interesting paths. I remembered my mother talking about a twin I was supposed to have had. Apparently after my mother birthed me and the placenta, the doctor noticed a twin had been growing along side of me. It didn't end up developing correctly and was reabsorbed into her body, and probably mine. The phenomenon is called "vanishing twin" and is pretty common.

I thought maybe I had some sort of spiritual connection with this vanished twin and that maybe contributed to my health problems. Could something that happened while in the womb affect my physical condition all these years later? Was the spirit of this twin energetically hanging on? Maybe some unspoken agreement I had made that I was now violating? Unspoken grief of my mother that I had accumulated inside?

One day, during an appointment with my acupuncturist, I brought the vanishing twin idea up. He was a pretty spiritual guy, and suggested I reach out to this twin spirit in some way. He advised me to ask the twin to meet me in a dream. Maybe I could discover something from this connection? I'm not religious, though I am spiritual and open to the mysterious of the universe. Maybe this plan had merit.

Making Contact

At that point in my healing journey, I was willing to basically try anything, so even though I have never tried to contact a spirit before, I decide to reach out to this twin spirit of mine. I went home and I took out a special pendulum I had acquired years earlier. I had some experience working with pendulums before and thought it might be a good way to try and communicate with the spirit. Whether there's actually a spirit there talking back I don't know, but pendulums always give an answer. The answers the pendulum gave to my questions this time confirmed a meeting with my twin sprit to be convened in my dreams that night.

I went to bed that evening like any other night and fell sleep. In the middle of the night I woke up with a start. The sound of barking dogs echoed across the ridge where I lived. Outside all the neighbor's motion lights were on. I felt a strange chill in the air although it was summertime.

It felt like the air was vibrating around me. My heart was racing and my skin pricked with goose bumps all of a sudden. I felt scared.

Is there some sort of spirit here right now? This doesn't feel right, I thought to myself.

"Not like this! Go away!" I yelled into the air.

Was this the twin coming to talk to me? In a dream I could handle it, but not this. This felt too real, too intense and I was not ready. I didn't know if it was all my imagination or not. After that experience, I decided I was not equipped to navigate the realms of communing with spirits. I decided to no longer pursue my twin's spirit and move to other mysterious pathways in the maze of my healing journey.

The Wise Healer

Many months later, I found myself at a nature awareness retreat. This was a gathering of folks learning about indigenous ways of education and practices connecting with the Earth, tracking animals, bird language, and peacemaking strategies.

One day, walking by the house where some of the facilitators were staying, I noticed one of our mentors, a Hawaiian medicine man named Kalani Souza, playing his ukulele. I had really enjoyed everything he had shared in the program and felt affinity with him. I began to walk away and was struck by a notion. In that moment, I felt this man might help me connect with my twin spirit. I hadn't thought about the twin in months but now I was compelled to share my story with Kalani. I walked into the house, and he stopped playing his ukulele looking up at me. I asked him if he had a moment, and told him I had been going through a tough time and was hoping for some advice. He looked into my eyes and became intensely present with me. He offered me a seat and an open heart to listen to what I had to say.

I shared with him what was going on for me physically, the challenges with my mother, and the question I had about my twin. The first thing Kalani did was validate everything I shared. That kind of validation was not a common experience for me growing up. The validation itself relaxed my whole being. Just to be fully heard is powerful healing. Kalani and I cried and embraced together like brothers.

I couldn't believe the presence and compassion he showed me. He and his wife Julie, an incredible healer and body worker herself, offered me a healing session that evening. Sunrise and sunset are spiritually reverent times of the day in native Hawaiian culture. Kalani's plan was to do a healing ritual while Julie did physical work on my body.

At sundown we set up the healing space. Kalani called to four directions and made offerings of saltwater. I stretched out on the table and Julie began working my muscles and manipulating my tense body. Kalani sang songs during the whole session. I didn't know it then, but it was the beginning of a great awakening.

The Dream of Death

The night of this first healing session happened to be a powerful cosmological event. It was Rosh Hashanah, the Jewish New Year, a full moon lunar eclipse, and the autumn equinox. Cosmological power was lined up and as I went to sleep I was not expecting to have this insightful dream:

I was in the middle of a huge fight. The place felt like the parking lot of the supermarket my mother shopped at. The scene was violent. There were men all around me, kicking and slashing with knives. I found myself fighting for my life. I didn't know why I was there or the people I was fighting. All I knew was I had to protect myself.

The battle seemed to go on for ages, although it was only a couple of minutes. I was scared and exhausted. As if to answer my fear, out of nowhere someone threw a knife directly into my heart. I fell to the ground. I could feel my life slipping away as I became disoriented. Blood was pouring out of my chest. I knew I was going to die. I don't know how I got here, or why this was happening but it was the end.

I woke up in bed with this dream still unraveling. I thought I was dead! I immediately burst into tears grateful to be alive. My wife woke up next to me and I shared the dream with her. I'd never felt the oncoming of death like that before. Somehow I knew it was more than just a dream. I knew some part of me was shedding away.

The next day, upon returning to the program, I went to find Kalani and told him my dream. He listened intently, then simply said, "I think you're ready now. Tomorrow we will take you into the teepee for a healing ceremony."

The Healing Ritual

The next day, I met with Kalani, Julie, my close friend Penny and a friend Kalani had asked to join. I don't remember her name, but she made up the fourth person to participate in this healing with me. Kalani began the ceremony in his traditional way of using saltwater to cast his circle and calling to the four directions. We went inside the teepee. I was asked to lie down on the ground in the middle. Kalani and the other three stood in each one of the four directions. Each one anchored a direction and together they formed a circle around me.

Kalani began to sing in his native language. Every now and then he would stop and ask me questions. I had no idea what was going to happen but I surrendered to the process. He began to call the spirit of my vanished twin into the circle. As we began to commune with this twin spirit, I had a sudden epiphany.

I had a flash of understanding that the spirit of this twin and I had made an arrangement when in the womb of our mother. Only one could survive and we agreed I was the one to be born that time. There was no need for me to feel guilty about it. It was a mutual agreement. These were startling thoughts that came into my head. The next epiphany was even more startling. This one was realized through a clue my mother had been telling me my entire life. If both of us had been born, I knew what my twins name would have been!

My Twins Name

My mother liked to tell me how she wanted to name me something other than Erik. She would tell me that the name Erik was what my father wanted. She apparently had another name she preferred. I never understood why she told this to me. I would think, "But my name is Erik so why does this matter?" Just one week before this healing ceremony she had brought this up again. She told me how she wanted to name me Zacharias.

Zacharias ... That could've been my twin's name! For some reason, this realization transformed some deep-held grief living inside of me. I didn't even know it was there, but I could feel it let go and alter in the moment. By the end of the ceremony I felt like a different person. I felt like I had healed an important relationship in my life. I understood myself better. I understood my mother better too, as I could see now the grief she still held from the birth of one, not two babies on the day I came into this world.

After the ritual I felt better than I had in years. I felt at peace. I felt present. In fact, twenty minutes after the ritual ended, a friend looked at me in surprise and said, "What happened to you? You look like you're ten years younger or something. You seem to be glowing." I was glowing and I was profoundly grateful. Grateful to Kalani and the community for helping me. Grateful to be held so safely through such uncharted and scary waters of my life. Grateful for the new understanding with my vanished twin. Grateful to feel so loved.

The Practice of Gratitude

In the busy culture we live in today, it can seem like an endless battle to barely stay ahead of our tasks. Once we accomplish one task, we instantly move to the next one. Our goals seem constantly out of reach and the cycle continues over and over again. What happens when we take a real break and stop our obsessive doing? What happens when we take a moment to check in with our accomplishments?

Can you see the beauty of your life when you slow down? Can you acknowledge the milestones you sped past? Do you see the love in your relationships? If you do, you are experiencing the feeling of gratitude. Are you able to take this action and acknowledge the blessing in your life? What does this experience feel like for you?

When you are grateful, you awaken joy in your heart and you can do this anytime. Practicing gratitude is a simple and nourishing action you can take at any moment. As humans, we easily focus on the negative in our life situations, but what happens when you focus on the positive? The activation of Joy is what's possible. The awareness of gratitude. Gratitude for your body, for good food, for friendship, for those who love you and the beauty of the Earth. Gratitude is medicine.

Some of you might be wondering, as I once did, how you can be grateful when your life is fraught with negative experiences. A life filled with trauma, illness, loss—what is there to be grateful for? Gratitude under these circumstances requires a surrendered mind.

Gratitude from the Pain

An advanced practice of gratitude is being grateful for the things causing you suffering and pain. This is daunting because our beliefs and programmed thinking reminds us how terrible our suffering is. In these agitated situations, surrender is the key to unlock the door of gratitude. With surrender, your mind can find clarity. You can now integrate the feedback your hardship is trying to point out to you. A lesson or gift can then be revealed. You may find the situation is not as bad as it seems. You may even be inspired by new solutions you didn't realize were there the whole time. Or, you may come to the realization that a major change is needed for your life to thrive. Gratitude can open these doors.

I discovered an amazing technique to be in gratitude all day long. The solution came from an unexpected place. Living with a chronic nervous system issue guided me to the solution. I had to learn to practice the art of gratitude while simultaneously being uncomfortable. Since gratitude and awareness go hand in hand, a disciplined routine of gratitude provided me with a well of peaceful awareness to fill my days. These reminders help to keep me present to my own capacity for joy and ease my self-inflicted suffering. Read on to learn how my practice was developed.

A practice of gratitude wakes you up to your patterns of painful thinking and painful doing. This works even in the most acute circumstances. With my physical condition, I'm constantly clenching the muscles in my body. My symptoms stem from this relentless tension. Over years of this pattern, new symptoms and issues arose out of the cumulative effect of straining my body for such a long time.

Moment to Moment

While on my healing journey I was encouraged to start a moment-to-moment relaxation exercise. This practice is based on awareness of each moment. Any moment I can, I consciously relax all the muscles in my body. This is a hard to remember to do. It was suggested I use a reminder buzzer to achieve moment-to-moment relaxation. This is the same technique folks with Temporomandibular Joint Dysfunction (TMJ) use to relax tension in their jaw muscles.

My condition is actually referred to as TMJ of the pelvis, so this treatment seemed like sound advice. I got myself a buzzer and set it to go off a few times per hour. This worked pretty well. Each time the buzzer vibrated I relaxed the tension in my body. Sometimes though, I was so focused on what I was doing, I wouldn't even feel the buzzer going off. For a time, I worried about missing these buzzer reminders. My worry about doing it wrong would then fuel my tension and anxiety, leaving me frustrated that the system was not working.

One day I had an epiphany. I decided that every time I thought about the buzzer (even if it wasn't going off), I would treat these thoughts as if the buzzer was vibrating. This began my new routine. Anytime I thought about the buzzer, whether it went off or not, I would relax the muscles in my body. This worked wonders on my mood and relieved my anxiety and some of my symptoms. After a year of practicing this moment-to-moment rhythm, I took it a huge step further. I included a powerful gratitude practice into my moment-to-moment relaxation.

Now when one of my reminder bells goes off, not only do I relax my tension, but I also intentionally feel gratitude for something in my life. I drop in, with intention, and give profound thanks. The practice of gratitude is a practice of healing, of loving, of recognizing and appreciating the gifts of this world. It has become one of the most powerful tools for activating my joy.

See the beauty in everything, and take the ninth mission ...

Mission: Practice of Gratitude
Go to Page 196

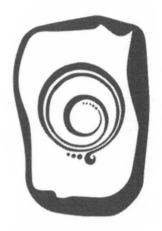

Three Levels
1. Personal Gratitude Statement
2. Share Gratitude
3. Gratitude for Challenges

PART FOUR: REGENERATION

As your mind gets clear and is calm,
You awaken to the thoughts that cause harm.
All that's left is love, joy, and peace;
Your dreams grow with these fertile seeds.

CHAPTER 11
PATTERNS OF NATURAL POWER

"To walk in nature is to witness a thousand miracles."
—Mary Davis

Humans are Nature

You are nature. You are made of the same energy as stars and planets. You are the breath of trees and waters of a deep ocean. This is not a theory, not a slogan, but scientific fact. The same water we drink, eventually becoming the liquid in our bodies, is the same water that has been on Earth since its formation as a planet. While some of Earth's water may have been seeded by comets, researchers from the University of Hawaii have concluded the origin of Earth's water came from its native planetary material. This water has continuously cycled through oceans and rivers, aquifers and lakes and every life form over the approximate 4.8 billions of years of our planets existence. You are 75 percent water.

Focus on your breath, drink a glass of water or take a bite of food. With these simple everyday actions, you experience your unbreakable bond with the natural world.

Did you know, all the air on the planet is made up of the same oxygen, hydrogen and carbon molecules that have been on Earth since its beginning? Biologists have confirmed, we are literally breathing the same air as our ancestors, the same air as the dinosaurs and the same air as the first red-blooded animals to be born from the sea.

Plant life and human life are closely akin to each other as well. We are connected in so many ways, even through the cells of our bodies. The chlorophyll molecule is almost exactly the same as the hemoglobin molecule of our blood cells. Both molecules have the exact same combination of oxygen, carbon, nitrogen, and hydrogen. The only difference is that chlorophyll has an addition of magnesium whereas hemoglobin has iron. That is right, the two molecules have only one compound different from each other! While they are structured differently, the similarities in composition are amazing!

Earth's Abundance

Our species is dependent on the life of this finite planet. We depend on the services of air-filtering forests, carbon-sequestering oceans and nutrient-developing soil bacteria. Looking to nature, we can see miracles happening every single day with little effort. Most of the time, nature works its miracles in slow deliberate cycles through symbiotic relationships and support systems. The Earth is truly abundant, providing everything we need to sustain thriving communities and societies.

Living close to the land can inspire our joy, creativity and generosity. Natural systems are built on exchanges of energy, cycles of life and death, and interdependent relationships. Humans can function like this too. It is wired already in our bodies and in our hearts. In the modern world, many have forgotten this great truth of who and what we are, but as we collectively remember and return to living close to the land, we will find a gentler, more satisfying, healthier way to live.

We can take our cues for action from the miracle of nature itself. The tree, the flower, the bird, they all teach us about beauty, patience, creation and love. The nurturing side of nature can give you pure love and you have that capacity too. You can spread that love like seeds on the wind.

Work Within Succession

Nature provides us with a blueprint for creation. A set of patterns for how to make change, grow abundance and develop masterful creations. One pattern we can use immediately in our planning and implementation is the process of succession. In nature, all systems evolve through succession. This is the process by which conditions slowly change over time due to newly emerging and complex systems. A mature forest provides a good example for this pattern.

How does a mature forest arrive at maturity? Does it spring out of nothing? Depending on the climate and location in the world, the succession story will be different. For many ecosystems, fire may have been a starting point. Let's start with the example of a fire-prone ecosystem to understand how succession works.

The Pioneers

Imagine a raging wildfire has burned through an environment. Many of the trees have been lost and the plants on the surface of the ground have been burned off as well. It looks like a desolate wasteland. Black and charred, the first the rains come and luckily seeds and roots survived the fire. First grasses, forbs and wildflowers will quickly cover the ground to protect it. In ecology we often call these "pioneers plants" as they are the first to emerge after a catastrophe. They are the first succession ...

The Second Succession

These pioneer plants attract a plethora of wildlife to graze, browse, pollinate and seek shelter in the first succession of plants after the fire. These creatures are nature's very own gardeners, moving seed and fertilizers around the ecosystem. Many birds carry shrub and tree seeds to the burned lands and plant them there. Now the second succession (we might call it the chaparral phase) in our forest story begins. Shrubs and small trees, planted by wildlife, spring up among the pioneer grasses on other plants.

These larger plant systems begin to change the soil, cast shade and create shelter for even larger animals. Small, young trees can find support from fast growing shrubs, giving the trees protection to establish.

Growing Strong

The third succession begins as small trees grow up and shade out grasses and shrubs. These trees create an even more robust wildlife habitat. The emerging forest now covers so much surface area that entire wildlife communities start to form on the canopy of these trees. Where I come from this would be a "woodland" phase. This young forest, often filled with a large diversity of trees species, provides necessary shelter for long-lived, slower growing trees to establish. Overtime, these long-lived trees eventually dominate the entire forest, shading out the first trees to grow from the second succession. This brings on the final succession, the climax forest.

The Climax Ecosystem

Once long-lived trees dominate a system, it can stay like that for thousands of years. This whole process of evolved succession may have taken hundreds of years to go from fire to mature forest. Each succession sets up conditions for the next succession to grow.

The Power of Working Within Successions

What does this have to do with you, right? The power of understanding succession is the power you can use to manifest your bold vision. Knowing that each milestone needs to first have the right foundation developed will aid you in your efforts. Reflect on how everything in your life has come through a process of succession. Think back to the biggest events that happened, whether good or bad. Usually you will be able to see some kind of buildup, a succession of growth or disturbance that enabled these events to occur.

Occasionally it's a short build up, at times it's many, many years of cumulative thinking and action leading to a major life change. You are a product of natural succession. It is how the universe operates. You can fight against it to your detriment or use this understanding as a vital tool towards living your life. Embrace these patterns of nature and use them for your own success.

Transforming yourself and how you function in the world can be a daunting task, but working with successions and phasing can help. The challenge of setting powerful goals, and the struggle to meet them in the timeframe you hope for, can be disappointing. Not achieving goals at all can leave you feeling exhausted and possibly even worthless. There's a story a lot of us tell ourselves when we perceive failure—it must mean we are unworthy, unaccomplished, a failure? Then anxiety and frustration can set in, leading to resentment. Don't fret, it may just be nature signaling to you that a different path is more aligned with your nature. Working and utilizing natural patterns like succession can lead you to awaken effective, stimulating and powerful creation powers of your life visions.

Instant Gratification

The big problem with current human thinking is the need for instant gratification. We set ourselves up for failure by boxing in our goals with unrealistic timelines. When we don't achieve our visions within these timeframes, we think our efforts have been in vain. The good news is we can change this limited way of thinking. Looking to patterns in nature, we find the most efficient and effective means of change and growth. Applying these patterns to our own efforts garner incredible results. The truth is, humans are natural beings, and we have within us the ability to operate like larger natural systems do. It is time we as a species utilize these powers and create a thriving Earth, both for humans and all of life on the planet.

Modern western civilization seems to have run away from our connection to nature. We consider the mind of humans to be a more powerful tool of change than ways of the Earth. We have believed this story to our own detriment. Yes, humans have built incredible civilizations and modern technological advances, representing miracles of human ingenuity. But at what cost? How many people are actually living joyful lives? How healthy are our communities? How healthy are our environments? What would happen if we joined forces with the power of nature? What would happen if we used the mind of humans to regenerate our communities and environments? What would humanity be if we chose Joy as the frame of success? Health and happiness being our economic indicators, rather than wealth in the form of money? If we did this, I think the world would enter an age of peace and prosperity.

Now is time for a bold new vision. To save our humanity, and activate our joy in regenerating our planet. Working against the flow of nature will not work for very long. Don't fight the tempest. Become the tempest. Fully align your thinking and actions with the natural successions of life and you will be unstoppable.

The Beauty in Everything

The longer you practice connecting to the present moment, the more beauty you see in the world. In your own house even, you may look at the shape of a table or the pattern on the wood and feel gratitude for its function and its beauty.

Perceiving the beauty in everything is the best technique for living joyfully all of the time. With this frame of seeing the world, everything you see or touch can bring joy to your heart as you feel light and at peace. There is no discovery or journey necessary for this practice. You can only perceive beauty in the present moment, so it is accessible to you at all times. Put the book down and appreciate the beauty all around you now.

Connecting with patterns in Nature can inspire you to experience beauty and the joy it inspires. Walk outside and feel the warmth of the sun. You may notice the trees swaying in the breeze. Or see moss-covered boulders and rejoice in their colors and textures. See how the water caressing the ground and nourishes life everywhere it travels. Listen to morning bird song and the diverse and beautiful melodies they express. Everywhere in nature is miracle of beauty and of connection. Nature is a web of loving relationships. Yes, there is violence and death in nature but it comes as part of an abundant cycle of life and connection. The connection we see in nature are the foundation for resilience and growth. We humans can learn much from observing the interactions of plants animals and elements. If we could remember that we too are nature, we may be able to model these forms of relationships in our own lives and in the design of our settlements and cultures.

Humans Are Beautiful Nature

Talk to other humans as we are all patterns of nature as well. Notice how beautiful every person is. Tap into your compassion for them, and the kindred, loving connection that is possible from human to human.

The practice of recognizing beauty has the power to thwart negatively escalating emotions. In moments when anger or fear gripped my emotions, I have found safe haven in the beauty of the world. A moment of breathing and the sound of birdcalls awaken me from my painful thinking. The taste of fresh fruit, the smell of a fragrant flower reminds me of what really matters. Reminds me of my place in the web of nature.

The embrace of the soft ground and the feel of rich soil in my hands reminds me of what sustains me. This is how we remind ourselves of our connection to divine energy, and our oneness with nature. Suddenly those negative thought patterns have no sway. They are petty, ego-driven, spreading unhealthy emotional pollen into the world. The gratitude of beauty brings a smile to my lips and I laugh out loud in the pure mesmerized joy of our planet. This part of the world, any of us can see any time if we choose to look. To see beauty is so easy. To be nature is so intuitive. So simple it fills me with love.

Because you deserve to be happy, take the tenth mission ...

Mission: The Happiness Mission
Go to Page 200

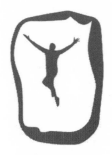

Three Levels

1. Day of Happiness
2. Week of Joy
3. Month of Bliss

CHAPTER 12

HEAR YOUR BODY

"New beginnings are often disguised as painful endings."
—Lao Tzu

Your body is one of the greatest gifts you have. While our bodies can cause us pain and suffering, they also provide sustenance and can give us immense pleasure. The human body is a miracle like all of nature. In today's fast-paced societies, many of us don't honor the role our bodies play in our daily lives. Often we sedate our bodies for the pleasure feeling and to dull any discomfort.

We have become so good at dulling our pain, we can go years and even whole lifetimes without truly listening to what our bodies are communicating to us. For many, it takes a physical crisis to wake up to those body whispers. Once you are awake to what the body is telling you, a life transforming process may unfold. The more you listen and follow the body's cues, the more your life begins to align with ultimate health.

The Signals of My Body

For myself, the signals my body gave me catalyzed some of my greatest lifelong lessons, ultimately leading to a more carefree and happy life.

What is your body saying to you? Your body is talking to you all the time. Is it telling you to sleep more? Drink more water? Stretch and move more? Does your body cause pain or strange sensations that can't be explained? These sensations can be scary. So scary, but, by being present to the body's needs, feeding it compassion and love, you will be guided in the right direction. Sometimes the signals of your body lead you to small changes and sometimes it can lead to major life changes.

Your body may even be telling you it's time to change careers, get out of a relationship, or take another kind of bold action. What really holds you back from taking guidance from your physical messages? I think most of us know deep down when we are out of alignment with our bodies. Our minds send us one direction while our body pleads to go another.

After many years of practicing body awareness, I realized my body was telling me to make sweeping changes in my life. Up until then I listened only to my mind. My thoughts had me spellbound to one way of thinking and I paid no attention to the signals of my physical state even though it was crying out for attention.

Anger at My Body

In fact, a lot of the time I was angry with my body and its discomfort. I would feel resentful for how it held me back from my aspirations. I would say to myself and others, *when my body is better, I'll be able to do all these greats things.* Achieve *all these huge goals.* Once I started to listen and finally take the actions my body led me to, I realized my mind may have been leading me astray. Maybe my body knew what is best for me after all.

Of course, like so many of us, I didn't choose to listen to the body. It forced me to pay attention. Funny how the body can do that sometimes. I was forced to listen and as I bent to the will of my physical needs, a beautiful path unfolded before me. Next thing I knew I was healing emotional wounds along with physical ones. I learned tools to better my relationships and experience more joy in life. Many of the tools shared in this book were born out of my personal healing journey. All the transformational missions were thrust upon me in the uncharted course of my life and the revelations my body led me to.

The Surrender

I surrendered to my body, listened and took action on its messages. I listened to the signals and followed the path they illuminated. Amazing experiences and opportunities began presenting themselves. The act of writing this book is a result of listening to my body. I felt compelled to write for many years but told myself I would never have time nor be a good enough writer. I still sensed writing my stories would be an incredible healing process for myself, and possibly others.

I also knew I couldn't maintain the outward expression of energy: managing, designing, teaching and facilitating teams of people and projects. My body was screaming for justice, for a different pace, a different environment. Burned out from many years of running a contracting company, launching new businesses, and teaching educational programs, I finally had the courage to give myself a sabbatical to recharge and write this book. This is an insightful turning point in my life.

Listening to our bodies is a key opportunity towards activating our Joy even when scary events happen. Our bodies know what they are doing. Crisis in our bodies may still arise. It can be difficult, but whatever is happening, have trust, listen, and align your life with the needs of your body.

The Snow Patch Incident

When I was sixteen years old I went on a backpacking trip with my dad and my brother. It was a long drive, sitting in the front bench seat of a simple Ford Ranger. As the youngest and smallest I sat in the middle between these two important men in my life. My dad didn't have a stereo in his car, so it provided an opportunity for conversation and bonding between us all.

After a long stretch on a major freeway, followed by long winding desolate roads, we made it to the trailhead nestled deep in the mountains. We grabbed our gear and started down the trail. The first campsite wasn't a far hike from the trailhead, nor was the peak of the tallest mountain in this part of California. We decided to "bag the peak" of the mountaintop before heading to our campsite for the night.

It was glorious and beautiful. Not another person for miles, just us and the pine trees, black bears, birds and mountain streams. A couple miles down the trail we saw the mountaintop in sight. After an easy climb, we reached the mountain's peak and the stunning views that came with it. I remember looking east and seeing thunderstorms in the distance, filled with lightning. Luckily, the storm was miles in the distance and moving away from us. After spending time enjoying these delights, we headed back to our campsite as dusk approached.

A Fun Idea

On our way down the mountain, we came upon a large snow patch. Most of the snow was melted this time of year, so finding a snow patch was an exciting treasure. My dad had a fun idea of sliding down the snow on our backsides from the top of the snow patch to bottom. It looked steep but also super fun. I held my trepidation and waited to see how it went for my dad as he went down first. He slid straight down and was able to slow and gracefully stop at the edge where it turned from snow to rocks. He stood up joyful and beckoned my brother to go next.

My older brother went a little faster. When he met the end of the snow patch he had a little too much energy. He hadn't slowed enough and quickly had to stand up and sprint across the rocks in order not to crash into them. He stayed on his feet and stopped safely. Now it was my turn. I was scared because of how close my brother had come to falling on the rocks. I decided to use the approach I observed my dad using. He had put his heels into the snow to maintain control and slow down at the end.

I sat down on the snow and began sliding. It was exhilarating! As I sped down the mountainside, I was acutely aware of my speed and my goal was to stop completely before the snow ended. I put my heels in the snow like my dad had done to slow myself down. The snow was pretty icy this late in the season and slowing down wasn't as easy as my dad had made it look. Digging my heels in the snow, I accidentally spun myself around backwards unable to control my speed or direction. Snow and ice was spraying everywhere. This was a terrifying moment. I was sliding backwards, coming closer and closer to the rock edge.

Next thing I knew; I was at the edge of the snow sliding quickly into the rocky terrain. Slam! I crashed into a small boulder. It hurt, it hurt tremendously. My heart was racing as my dad and brother rushed to my aid. As I stood up, I exclaimed, "I think I broke my tailbone." My tailbone and lower spine area throbbed painfully. I took some time breathing through it. We had just spent the last seven hours getting to this point. It was the first day of our long anticipated backpack trip. Our first campsite was close by. What did I do now? Was my tailbone really broken or maybe just bruised? Did I treat this like an emergency and leave the trip immediately or go set up our camp? In that moment, I realized just how hungry and tired I was.

Being Stoic

I decided to try and walk it off. I didn't want to make us turn back, and although it was painful, I found I could still walk. I put my forty-pound backpack on and we hiked to the campsite. The next few days were pretty uncomfortable, we hiked multiple miles a day carrying our big packs. Sleeping on the hard ground and using only thin pads was difficult for my throbbing tailbone.

Although my backside was sore, I kept a good attitude. I enjoyed the beauty of the trip and the rare opportunity to be with my dad and brother for a few days of quality time together. It turned out to be a great trip with the exception of the snow patch incident.

After the backpack trip, I completely forgot about what happened on the slopes of those mountains ... Little did I know what a life altering experience it truly was.

The End of Comfort—Nine years after the snow patch incident

Nine years later, my life changed forever. I was at my mother's house and we had a sweet visit together. I was getting ready to drive the thirty minutes back to my home in the country. Right before I left, I had to use the bathroom. When I got out my mom was standing there with a worried look on her face. She said with concern, "Erik, are you okay?" I responded blankly, "Yeah, I'm totally fine, why?"

Apprehensively she said, "Well, do you realize you just had to pee three times in the last half hour? I've never seen you do that before." I thought about it, and realized I had gone to the bathroom a bunch of times since I had been at her house. I told her I felt fine but a glimmer of anxiety awoke inside. I said my goodbyes, got into my truck and started driving home.

Ten minutes into the drive, I felt like I had to use the bathroom again. Again? Why did this feel so urgent? I wasn't sure I could hold it. My heart fluttered as I felt intense energy sweep through my body. What was going on? It was weird. I stopped off at a gas station and used the bathroom. From there I was able to drive the rest of the way home without having to stop again.

But later that day I found myself going to the bathroom again and again and again. That first flickering fear quickly turned into a knot of anxiety.

Was there something happening to me? The next few days and weeks became difficult as all comfort left my body. I found myself needing to use the bathroom repeatedly. I had a hard time driving even a short fifteen minutes to the closest main town. I had to start canceling my meetings and step away from some of my projects as I was having a hard time traveling anywhere.

Humbled

Constantly feeling the need to use the bathroom is a humbling experience. I would never feel relief when I went, so I was in a perpetual state of discomfort. My constant fear gripped me and I started to have almost daily panic attacks. The attacks came on urgently and with ferocious intensity. This was a distressing time of my life.

If I couldn't find a place to relieve myself fast enough, the energy inside my body went up into my throat and I would find myself gagging and dry heaving. After a couple of these experiences in the car and in public, a deep fear set in. I became scared of going into public places. I had to quit many of my projects that generated my main source of income. I had to stop teaching and traveling and therefore couldn't participate in the activist campaigns or design course that I organized and fundraised for. This was the beginning of the next part of my life ... Ups and downs, highs and lows, all centered around dealing with the physical and mental symptoms of this new phenomenon happening in my body.

11 Years Later—A Post to Social Media

Eleven years after the fateful day at mother's house when comfort left my body, a turning point occurred. A new revelation presented itself and it changed everything ... Below is a post I made to social media about this turning point in the maze of experiences healing myself. Writing this post was an act of healing in of itself. I kept my physical issues mostly to myself and many friends and colleagues didn't realize what an impact it had in my daily life. It was a moment of vulnerability, I could see a new era on the other side of this and the message I wrote for the world, was the seed of a new frame to seeing my health, a new narrative and a new freedom:

The following is a rare personal post on my part. I appreciate anyone reading this long story you are witness to. My true intention for writing this is so I can hear it myself. So I can let go and create a new healthy path for myself. I realize if I can't believe I can heal then I never will. I now believe.

I'm calling in my ancestors to help me ... I'm inviting deep healing and the shedding of all the obstacles holding me back. Most people don't know for the last eleven years I've been living with a nervous system dysfunction I plan my life around. I wasn't ever properly diagnosed and after a dozen doctors, acupuncturists, diet changes, physical therapies, shamanic rituals, herbalism, and numerous other strategies I never managed to heal myself.

All of those healing experiences changed me in profound ways and long ago I came to terms with my condition as one of the BEST things to ever happen to me. It is because of this healing journey, I was unleashed in the world the way I am now. Through all of the last decade, no matter what was going on it has always been a physical and mental struggle to keep going and I always knew I was only functioning at maybe 60 to 70 percent of my capabilities.

I always tell myself I have enough health to be happy and productive and even though I'm constantly uncomfortable I keep being grateful for everything and everyone in my life and the opportunities that have been given to me. Every now and then I go back into the deep dark depression that so marked the first two years of being sick and my coping abilities erode away for a time.

Every time this has happened I try to get back to my "therapies" and I once again search for "solutions" and try to diagnose the "problem." Each time I end up flaring the symptoms up too much and get even more depressed and give up ... again ... Be grateful for what I have, keep going, I have an amazing life, I'm full of love, it's okay ... life goes on ...

In over a decade of these cycles I never have been able to shake this thing. It has literally ruled me and my family's life. Chronic issues can be very hard on families. I'm so grateful for the unconditional and enduring support my wife Lauren Ohlsen and my two children have given and give me every day. My kids have never known me otherwise so for them this is how Dad is. I do not want this for my family anymore.

The thing about a chronic illness or pattern is after a while you learn to live with it and you do your best to function and live a happy life. You integrate "tools" to help you cope with normal day-to-day stuff and you prepare and plan to avoid traumatic experiences during days when you want to make big accomplishments.

I have often wondered though, what it would be to feel comfortable and have normal bodily functioning again. I often look out and notice how almost everyone around me doesn't worry so much about needing to go to the bathroom all time, like I do. I'm sad people have to wait for me all the time. I'm embarrassed every time I have to interrupt a meeting I'm in so I can again use the bathroom.

I'm devastated when I can't leave a situation or I'm stuck in the car and can't get to a bathroom. Those times I usually end up in a full blown panic attack, dry heaving, gagging and heart racing. Those are tough days and although it used to be daily, the panic attack experiences happen once every few months now.

The reason I share this story now is because a breakthrough has recently happened. For the past three years I haven't tried to get help at all. I gave up on healing myself and therefore have been coping and getting by. Then a few weeks ago my wife referred me to a health care provider named Jeannie Kerrigan, she thought I should go see. I've been exhausting my coping abilities recently anyway and thought I should go see what this new provider had to offer.

One of the main things Jeannie does is focus on the nervous systems and specifically does work on a nerve bundle behind the tailbone called the ganglion of impar ...

Here is what happened:

On my second visit as I'm stretched out on the table, she went for this nerve bundle and made a discovery exclaiming: "Oh my, Erik, it looks like at some point in your life your tailbone must have been crushed. It's smashed in, pinching your nerves back there ..."

"What!!! My tailbone crushed at some point in my life?? Pinching nerves at the base of my spine??" I thought.

In the moment I remembered a time when I was 16 years old sliding down a snow patch ... [here I recounted the snow patch incident in the social media post. I will spare those details again!]

When I research what to do about a broken tailbone it is basically deal with it or get surgery. Surgery has a minimum one-year recovery time and in many cases because there are so many muscles and nerves attached to your tailbone it doesn't always actually fix the problem. So surgery is completely out for me. There is one more option and lucky for me, Jeannie, the amazing healer I just saw, has done it numerous times before in her thirty years of experience.

Starting today and then twice more this week she is going to relax the muscles around my tailbone and see if she can pull it back a small amount. She is going to focus on getting to the nerve bundle behind the broken and now fused tailbone and see if she can relieve some of the pressure on the nerves. Pull the bone back a little and relieve the pressure on the nerves. Tailbones are one of those bones designed to have a little flexibility and we are counting on my body to cooperate with this. I'm very optimistic!

I already had my session today and it was incredibly painful but feels okay now. Since then I've been having massive emotional releases as so much of the trauma we humans experience in life gets stored in our nervous system. I haven't had this level of emotional release since my mom died a few years ago. In fact, I see her face in my mind's eye right now and all afternoon since my session. This Friday and Saturday I get the last two sessions for this round and she is going to go deeper each time. I'm nervous about what is going to happen but I'm ready. I'm ready to move on with my life. I'm ready for my body to function normally again. I'm ready to not be held back any longer.

I'm ready for this burden to be lifted from the shoulders of my family. For me this marks a time in my life where for the first time in a long time I will once again seize fully my own strength and power. Sky's the limit. The next era of my life begins. This story as written, will be the last time I write about it with this intention. The whole point of writing this is to get it out of my body. I'm moving on from this now. Thank you for witnessing. This week ahead will be my shedding and on the other side my wings will fly ... Blessed be."

Make your own self-care plan, take the eleventh mission ...

Mission: Heal Your Body Mission
Go to Page 203

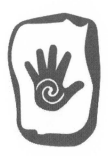

Three Levels

1. Gift for Your Body
2. Create A Self-Care
3. Make A Commitment

CHAPTER 13
NATURE TENDING NATURE

"Even after all this time the Sun never says to the Earth, 'You owe me.' Look what happens with a love like that. It lights up the whole sky."
—Hafiz

What if you could be as strong as a mountain? What if you were as flexible as water? As lighthearted as air? What if you could harness the power of the Sun and turn it into life, just like plants and trees? If you could do these things you would be unstoppable in generating abundance, happiness and love throughout your world.

The truth is, you can harness these powers. You are abundance. You are nature. You have the pattern of the universe inside of you. When you realize that you are a strand in the web of life, you can harness the creation powers of the web itself. By continually opposing that connection we turn down the tap of universal energy. The more you remember these relationships, the more you find you can nurture the gifts nature provides us.

The human mind and body are simultaneously the most destructive and most effective tools for regenerating Earth's environments. You can nurture the soil and clean the water and plant trees. These are gifts you can give back to the web of life. And these gifts that you give, generate more miracles of nature as they grow, blossom, fruit and seed in their cycles. Generosity to nature is as necessary as generosity to your fellow humans. It is the gift you give your descendants. It is key to thriving future generations.

Tend to Nature

In this day and age, disconnection is more common than connection with the natural world. Humanity is driven by its technology, and we've drifted farther and farther away from being cultures that live in harmony with the land. But even within all of our technological advances of our modern-day world, every material item that we harvest, mine, build with, utilize or have in our lives comes from land. We cannot disconnect from the Earth in reality, only in the illusion of our minds. Instead of disconnected thinking, what would happen if we acknowledged and even invested in the connection to our home planet? What would humanity and the world look like if we celebrated and tended the land?

It may seem strange to talk about tending nature in a personal development book. But tending to nature is the same as tending to humans. Tending to humans is tending to yourself. And we want to utilize every possible avenue towards designing and living happy lives.

The simple act of planting a tree can have profound beneficial consequences over many years and even generations. This is why I've included a *Tend to Nature Mission* in this book. I feel it would be incomplete to remove nature from the focus of living joyful lives. To our modern world many people spend time in nature for enjoyment.

Working Close to The Land

Spending time in nature is great, but tending to the land—in a hands-on way—has incredible benefits for humans and the environment. In fact, the benefits can go way beyond a day-to-day benefit and can have lasting effects for generations. Watch what happens if you get your hands in the ground, even just a little bit. Be aware of how you feel when working closely with the land. The success of seeds sprouted by your own hand, or harvesting food from a plant that you've tended. These are yet more methods to ground your nervous system and connect with the present moment. To be of service to the beauty that surrounds you. To engage in the miracles of life. To tend to nature, is to be the miracle of life.

As a lifelong steward of the land, the hard work of repairing ecologies taught me so much about natural systems, plants, animals, fungi, climate, soils, cycles of birth and death and so much more. Truly, the education of the nature is life-long, never ending, and as we teach our young ones, it becomes a generational venture.

Committed to tending every landscape I had access to, I consistently built huge gardens in every place I lived, even when I was renting. It is probably common knowledge that not everyone is willing to invest into a rental living situation. Many landlord/tenant agreements forbid the tenant from changing the landscape. For those that allow it, and for folks who have the time and energy to do it, there is great opportunity in tending those rental landscapes. I jumped on it every chance I got.

In my experience, the abundance reciprocated from working the land to grow food or medicine, and create an enjoyable outdoor environment, vastly outweighs the ownership of that piece of ground. Every time I would leave a garden—moved to a new home—I would propagate all my favorite plants from the existing garden. Another beautiful cycle of nature: the ease by which we can propagate most plants. I would essentially leave a garden behind and take a garden with me to the next place. Every place I have lived became abundant with fresh healthy food to harvest every day. This is a legacy every human can contribute to for themselves and the planet.

Human Can Repair the Planet

Humans can be regenerative support systems for our environment. So much so, that we can even repair the most abused and destroyed landscapes. The industrial human era brought on a destruction of natural environments that continues to this day. And while humans created the mess, we are also best poised to regenerate this planet quickly and miraculously. The physical regeneration of landscapes is not very difficult as you will see in the story below. We have all the knowledge, principles and technology we need to make huge strides in regenerating the planet. It's the will of people to actually do it that poses the greatest obstacles. This is another reason I wrote this book, to activating the caring side, the loving side in us all. From there all healing is possible.

The first home I ever owned was nestled in a destroyed landscape. It was a third of an acre lot in the town where I live, Sebastopol, California. For at least twenty years prior to my family moving in, the soils were highly compacted and the parking area was directing rainwater right to the foundation of the house. I always love a challenge when designing landscapes, and this posed a beautiful challenge. A demonstration of what's possible. A model of restoring the urban environment. How quickly can we turn this parking lot into a lush, water harvesting, food producing, beautiful place for my family to grow up in?

We set to task and what we accomplished in that first year was empowering. We removed all the asphalt and concrete, we loosened the compacted soils, and consolidated the gravel into pathways and patios. Within two years the entire site was completely transformed. We designed our landscape to be a high functioning, water harvesting system. Due to runoff patterns of our neighbors, we were able to route, catch, and infiltrate over 400,000 gallons of rainwater every year in this landscape. We planted eighty-plus fruit and nut producing trees, which begin providing fresh harvests in year one and forever after. A diversity of insects, birds and other beneficial life made homes in our gardens, helping to manage pests and bringing birdsong and wonder to our space.

Return On Investment

In the five years we lived at this home, we gave dozens of tours and classes to over one thousand people from all over the world, visiting our region to learn about permaculture and ecological design. The site not only functioned as a demonstration of regenerating destroyed environments, but also an experiment in social organizing and community building. We created a co-housing community in our neighborhood by utilizing the paradise landscape we had built. Friends of ours who lived alongside the property removed fences and put in gates and we reveled together in the beauty of the ecological garden. We managed and harvested the yields of this system together.

The truth is, we can all participate in the regeneration of our landscapes. Not because it's trendy, progressive or anything ideological. Because to be on the land brings people joy. To harvest, work and celebrate together, provides benefits to our health, our stress levels and our sense of connection, to each other and with nature.

I have dozens of stories like the one above documenting the transformation of hundred-acre ranches, city halls, libraries, city blocks, schools and so on. There's an entire movement spreading like wildfire around the planet to regenerate our landscapes, and support and love one another. This movement can start in your own backyard even if it's just a windowsill. It can start by planting one seed and nurturing it to growth. It can start by joining one volunteer garden party, attending a farm to table celebration or any other opportunity to connect with the land. To connect with your community.

The land brings us together in profound ways. Nature is tending nature in this dynamic dance of connection. The nature of humans is tending the nature of the Earth. The nature of the Earth is tending the nature of humans. And so it has been since the beginning of life on the planet. Together in this way, people and the environment, we can all thrive, living lives rich in abundance. And ensure that our descendants, the generations ahead of us, our great-grandchildren's grandchildren, have the same opportunity to thrive on a healthy planet.

The Love of Nature

You were born perfect. You are made of the same energy and essence of nature. Inside of you lives the same energy that created the universe. Can you feel it? Go outside and look around. The interactions between water and topography, between birds and plants are all expressions of love. These are all woven of mutual relationship. Symbiotic gain. They are all dependent on each other, dancing in a master choreography of give and receive, birth and death. Every person on the planet is part of this web of relationships.

Nature loves you. Total, unconditional love. Nature gives you everything you need: water, food, shelter, medicine, clothing, recreation. It's a powerful act to recognize this love. The interconnectedness of nature—to which you are connected as well—serves as a beautiful and constant reminder of the love that exists in every moment on the planet today.

What if you tapped into this force? As you tap into it, what if you turn it on yourself? How would your life change if you gave yourself all the love in the world? All those times you tried so hard to impress someone to gain their love. All those times you went against your truth to be accepted by others? What if you gave that love and acceptance to yourself first and foremost?

As you become aware of the love inside, your interconnectedness with the love around you gets easier to connect with. Life has a bit more joy. The more you reside in this connection, the longer you hold space for this love to grow, the more you begin to transform. Without effort, you emanate this energy to the people around you and the love inside them recognizes it and reflects it back. Little by little, we end up helping each other live happier lives.

Returning to love is not so much a journey or a discovery, as it is an awareness of what's already there. Right now, behind your stories, your thoughts, and assumptions, is the full power of the universe. It is there always and will never go away. Access it to change your life and you will change the world.

Unconditional Love

To have unconditional love is to be at peace with yourself just the way you are right now. Peace within only comes from utter and total acceptance of who you are. This is unconditional love.

When you can love others unconditionally because you love yourself unconditionally, then no matter what anyone says or does, the grief and trauma of those words or actions cannot affect the peace inside you. Judgment of others dissolves as you accept people for who they are. It takes a strong sense of awareness to not get caught up in the games of people, but by being present to the love that is always there, it becomes easier to feel this compassion for others. With compassion you can begin to see people for who they truly are beneath their stories, words and actions.

This kind of love is rare in the modern-day culture and I myself can't say I've mastered this way of being. I can say that by applying the tools shared in this book, I now spend most of my time in this state and it is a blissful and successful approach to thrive.

Please always remember, your potential is limitless; your love lasts as long as time itself, your love is deeper than the deepest ocean and larger than the largest mountain. Your love is stronger than the densest steel and braver than the greatest warrior. Your love can never be taken away, it is always with you, and it's the gateway to your life purpose.

Your love is the special medicine you brought to the planet. It is the greatest gift you can give to yourself. It is the greatest gift you can give others. Your love heals the planet, your love is your home, your love is the real you. Give it to yourself and share it with the world.

The joy of nature awaits, take the twelfth mission ...

Mission: Tend to Nature
Go to Page 207

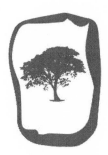

Three Levels
1. Plant a Tree and/or spend time in nature
2. Grow Your Own Food
3. Plan a Community Project

CONCLUSION

"Love is the great work though every heart is first an apprentice ... Happiness is the great work, though every heart must first become a student."

—Hafiz

Strands of Life, Weaving Together

This has been my story, my lessons, and my transformations—these are the strands of life I'm weaving together. I am in love with life, people, and the Earth and it's a wonder-filled existence. The four strategies of this book—Vision, Connection, Transformation and Regeneration—act as pillars for how I live my life.

Vision

Learning to live through the mind frame of Joy makes a happy life possible. Inspired by this positivity, I'm able to envision a bold life design and when it turns out differently than I had imagined ... I can accept the truth, adapt my vision to reality, and continue gratefully. All this while using my superpowers, my inherent gifts to stay creative, passionate and in touch with my true nature. This is honoring my true self and living limitlessly.

Connection

As an emotional pollinator, I know that the words and energy I share with others will affect them. Maybe even change them. That is why I have to cultivate an ability to be aware. With awareness of what's happening inside me and around me at all times, I can decipher my own truth from my own lies. This enables me to read the energy of those I connect with so I can communicate empathetically with them. As I become aware of my capacity for unconditional love, I share that with my community and my planet. I spread seeds of generosity that create peace and generate abundance.

I have seen what's possible when kindness and generosity are shared. I've experienced the gift of giving, whether it's feeding the hungry or building community gardens, lives were touched, even transformed. Generosity finds its place at the core of how I operate now, the positive energy it creates is too addictive, too mesmerizing. People want to feel loved by others. People yearn for connection and as emotional pollinators we can all make it happen.

Transformation

Does the grief in your life ever really go away? I don't think it disappears but transforms into something else. Maybe it transforms into gratitude? Maybe it transforms to forgiveness? Maybe it transformed into something negative, a heavy weight to carry around? I've carried plenty of these heavy stories and I'm always checking to see what's still latched on. These stories, as I know now, need to be faced. Every time I face them, it is a rite of passage. These rites of passage can be enlightening, full of emotional release, mental clarity and joyful promise.

"Why did I carry that around for so long?" I ask myself. Now I know. I don't need to live like that. I can transform this energy with my forgiveness. I can acknowledge it, accept it, even love it, with my gratitude. This is the healing of my body in action. This is the healing of my mind, and of my emotions.

With these tools and practices I can weather the storms of my life. I can plant seeds of forgiveness and gratitude in my community. I can authentically help others face their own fears and be free from the stories they're carrying. Transformation comes at a cost. Who you were before is not who you are after transformation is done with you. The fear of change is mighty, but it's the change that grows. It's the change from story to truth. The change from depression to happiness. From here, we all find our own special healing and awaken to a joy-filled life.

Regeneration

I am filled with optimism. Optimism about my own life and my own health. I'm optimistic about the future of my community and of our shared planet. Why am I so optimistic? At the time of writing this book, I'm still suffering from chronic discomfort. Many biological systems on the Earth are in peril, including human communities. People are at war; people are filled with hate. This hate that stems from so much pain, and the suppression of so much grief. What is optimistic about this situation? I will tell you ...

As I've learned in my life, we all have the power to regenerate. We can regenerate ecosystems. We can regenerate relationships. We can regenerate our own exhausted, stressed out, and broken bodies. This is a power we are all bestowed with. To use our love to regenerate everything around us. This is why I'm optimistic about things. Because, I think deep inside the true nature of every person, is a seed of love ready to sprout, to grow, and take root. My mission has become clear. It's time to water all these little seeds in everyone around me, all the time and do it with generosity, forgiveness, and gratitude. This I can do as an awake emotional pollinator. You can do this too.

We can regenerate in other ways to. Spending days close to nature, hands in the soil, seeds in hand, tending to that which gives life. The natural world. Nature gives life. In this way, we can regenerate the collective pain of current and past cultures at the same time. The disconnection we experience from our belief systems can be restored when we tend to our communities and environments. Our ancestors knew the way, and so do we. We can foster new cultural stories of regenerative connections to each other and the land. Let's regenerate that inherent connection of humans and their environments. Let's do it in community and rejoice in our common heritage as members of the Earth. As we nourish those seeds, we are nurturing a bright future for generations to come.

Unleash Your Power

Strip away everything you know and think. In this moment, strip away your story about yourself. Strip away your judgments about others. For a moment, stop worrying trying to please others. Strip away your biggest worries and allow your greatest fears to be put on hold. For a moment let it all go. What is left?

When you stop thinking, what is left? What is left when you are fully present? What is left when you stop believing your lies and assumptions? It's love. Love is left. Awareness of your body is left. Awareness of your surroundings, the Earth, other people, and awareness of what makes you happy. From this place you can solve problems. From this place you can make peace. From this place you can tap your creative potential. From here wounds are healed and forgiveness is given and received.

From here you can share your love with the world. You surrender to the present, to what's real. You find the courage that has always been there. The courage to stand up for your own happiness. Everything you need is inside you right now. The intellect, the talents, the time. It can be hard to believe. You may be reading this thinking, "How can this be? I still need to learn so much." Or, "For my vision to manifest there are many things I need to change my life."

Or you feel the trap of past trauma, or an illness, or an emotional obstacle. Do these beliefs really have to keep you from realizing your dreams? Maybe some of it is just the mind and the ego's way of tricking you. Keeping you trapped in cycles of grief and pain. Of course there's more to learn, of course there's more grief to be felt, but who you are is still all you need. Accept who you are. Rejoice in who you are! You are a gift to this world. Accept your life situation as your reality and surrender to the moment. This will wipe away the obstacles, thought patterns and behaviors that keep you from unleashing your superpowers to their fullest extent.

Activate Your Joy

Let your superpowers shine like the sun. Unleash the love inside and empower your dreams. Activate your life by design. Activate limitless thinking. In the end, it comes down to the simple fact that you are your only limitation. Your thought patterns, your beliefs, your attachments to your griefs, your grievances, your ideas about others, your need to be accepted, your goal of doing what others expect of you, these are the true obstacles in your way to a joyful, fulfilling and love filled life every day.

When you free yourself from the self-imposed restraints, the ripple effect in your life will be monumental. But you won't be worried about that because what will matter to you most is being true to your heart, giving justice to your body and enjoying the beauty of every moment. Are you still going to get upset? Still going to feel angry? Are difficult situations and things still going to happen?

Yes, all of these things will still happen, but you have the awareness of seeing them for what they are. All you have to do is accept yourself and those feelings, and do your best. Doing your best is all you need to do, no matter what happens. You will find the ability to judge yourself a little less every day and forgive a little more too. The integrity of your life, the dreams and ambitions that you hold, are all inside, not outside of you. Let it out! I know that it's scary, I know that people in your life may perceive you in a way that's uncomfortable. I know that the life you have now might unravel. But let it.

I invite you to let all that go. I invite you to stop listening to the judge that's inside. I invite you to not believe the stories about how much of a victim you are. Don't settle for what other people tell you. Don't settle for what your thoughts tell you and follow your intuition instead. I invite you to tap into the beauty, the superpowers and the gifts inside of you.

Do what is joyful and step on a path aligned with the universe. Opportunities will flourish, doors will open, and your relationships will transform. Doing this with present moment awareness, you will unleash your true power and activate joy everywhere. I support you to free yourself! No matter what has happened to you, no matter what your situation, if you choose a mission of Joy, you will find Love. True, unconditional love. Now and forever, drink deep of this love and be who you are meant to be.

Don't forget to claim your Activate Your Joy Life Design Playbook PDF
here! http://erikohlsen.com/ayj-playbook/

Join the Activate Your Joy Life Design Facebook Community here:
https://www.facebook.com/groups/184539945414028/?source=create_flow

PART FIVE:

12 POWERFUL MISSIONS TO

DESIGN A LIFE YOU LOVE

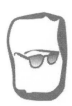 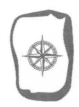

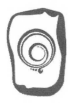   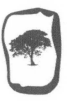

MISSION:
TRANSFORM YOUR FRAME OF MIND

The quest begins! The missions build on one another so make sure to do them in the presented sequence. As you take part in this exercise do not judge yourself by what you discover. The more truthful you are with yourself, the more powerful this mission will be. Don't fret the dark thoughts that may arise. This book will teach you step-by-step how to completely change your frame and guide you towards alignment with your dreams and happiness.

Your frame is the lens you see the world through. Many parts of who you are, your thoughts, stories, belief systems, and the grievances you carry all affect your frame. Go in fully and follow the mission all the way through to the end. You will love yourself for it. If you still feel unsettled after this mission, remember to be gentle with yourself. These missions build on one another. Be gentle and good luck! This is the beginning ...

Two Levels
1. Identify Your Current and Ideal Frame
2. Transform Your Frame of Mind

Tools and Practices:
- Mind Map
- Core Values Assessment
- Bullet Point Lists
- Creative Collage Scene

Level 1

Identify your Current and Ideal Frame

This is an important assessment of your current frame of thinking. Take the time to answers all the questions.

Step 1

Ask yourself the questions below and write down the answers. While you may feel the answers will vary depending on your mood, think in general terms when answering. Use bullet points for your answers to make this easy:

How do I feel like I'm being treated by others?
How do I want to be treated differently?
How do I treat others?
How do I want to treat others differently?
How do I treat myself?
How do I want to treat myself differently?

To make this assessment more relevant, ask yourself the above questions within different groups in your life. This will help you identify how your outward frame changes depending on which circle you are engaging in.

How do I want to be treated and how do I treat others in ...
My work and career?
My family?
My friendships?
My romantic relationship(s)?
My community?

Step 2

Read through a couple times and reflect on the answers to all these questions. Were there any general themes that came up? Do you find you hold yourself to the same standards as you hold others to? Write down any revelations you have through this process.

Level 2

Transform Your Frame

Did you attach yourself to any judgments that came up during Level 1? It is likely they will come up, and it's perfectly normal. Don't worry if your answers ended up positive or negative from your point of view. In this level, you have a chance to create an ideal frame for your life with intention.

Step 1

This step is all about brainstorming your ideal values and ways of thinking. There are a variety of different brainstorming techniques you can use for this process. If you have a process that works well for you, then please use that. Or you can create a mind map (preferred), a creative scene or collage, a bullet point list or whatever works for your learning style. Make sure to follow the link below to get a better understanding of how to use a mind map for your brainstorming process. http://erikohlsen.com/activate-your-joy-support/

Step 2

Once *Step 1* is complete, go back over your brainstorm with a focus on what kinds of patterns are repeating. Distill your brainstorm down by clumping together phrases, words and statements that are the same or similar. Once you make it through one time to distill your brainstorm, go back through once more and try to distill further.

Step 3

Your goal now is to take the distilled brainstorm and write five sentences from it. These value statements represent the essence of what your ideal frame is. These sentences will have to be as succinct as possible. Such as:

"I strive to treat others with the same respect and kindness I want to be treated with."

"I want to live in a home environment which is emotionally healthy, a place I can relax and rejuvenate and a place I can raise a healthy family."

"I will build a career grounded in the gifts and passions I have to share and in a work environment which values dignity, good communication, compassion, and productivity."

"When hard times or situations happen I will do my best not to react from fear. I will bring my love and awareness to the situation and do my best to contribute to solutions."

"I value humor in my life and work and will strive to create space for more laughter."

Step 4

Print your five sentences out and post them in places to remind yourself of them, such as your kitchen, car, on your smartphone, in your office, etc. Throughout the day, reference back to these statements as a source of inspiration and guidance towards cultivating your ideal frame of mind. This work takes a lot of practice and constant forgiveness of yourself and others as you dissolve your old way of looking at the world. Do your best and be patient with yourself.

MISSION:
AWAKEN YOUR SUPERPOWER

Time to activate your inherent superpowers in all aspects of your life. Don't hold back your gifts. Share them freely and transform your world. Galvanize these powers like you never have before. Recognize these as special gifts that come naturally to you. Discovering your superpower gifts is one of the first steps in the journey to living your life in truth and creating happiness in yourself and your community.

Three Levels
1. Power your Passions
2. Distill Your Superpowers
3. Superpower Activation

Tools and Practices:
- Non-Edited Brainstorm
- Mind Map
- Superpower Reminders
- Reflection journal (workbook)

Level 1

Power your Passions

Step 1

Write down a list of all the things that make you happy. This is a brainstorm so *do not edit* them during this exercise. Don't worry about whether you think something is possible or not. As you fill in the different categories with what makes you happy, focus on the behaviors, actions, or goals. Allow yourself to dabble in both present situations and experiences as well as goals for the future.

Step 2

Take your list and then put it into the following categories:
Hobbies:
Relationships:
Work/career:
Free time:

Level 2

Distill Your Superpowers

Step 1 (only step)

Distill your passions by similarity. The goal is to emerge with three core superpowers. For example, if you ended up with:

- I'm a good listener
- I value effective communication
- I'm good at offering feedback to people

You might distill this into one superpower—**Communication Power**

Level 3

Superpower Activation

Once you have completed Level 2, it is time to activate these superpowers like never before. This level is what it is all about. This level is almost like three levels in of itself. I would advise you start by spending one day to one week to complete each step of this level. Feel free to take as much time as you need.

Day/Week 1+

Step 1

Choose one of your superpowers to use on this day. Dedicate the day (or week) to this superpower. Make sure you start by choosing a day that represents a normal "work day" for you.

Step 2

Throughout the day you will use your superpower in as many situations as you can. Watch what happens.

Step 3

At the end of the day record one revelation you had. Did anything change for you? Anything surprising? What is your emotional state? Was this practice hard to implement or easy?

Day/Week 2+

Follow the same challenge described in *Day 1* with your second superpower. Make sure to record one major observation at the end of the day and reflect with the same questions.

Follow the same challenge described in *Day 1* with your third superpower. Make sure to record one major observation at the end of the day and reflect with the same questions.

Final challenge:

Use your superpowers to the fullest extent every single day and experience your world transforming.

MISSION:
DESIGN YOUR LIFE

Now to the drawing board! Time to design your dream life. Make sure you have read the *Dream Life by Design* chapter before starting this mission. There is important information there about the architecture of your plan and more. In this mission you will craft a new story for your life. How bold is your vision? Let this mission become your new life design plan. This is the recipe for creation. You are your own world creator. Create a world you love!

Five Levels
1. Map Your Dream Life
2. Develop Short and Long Term Goals
3. Dream Life Timeline (Reverse Engineering)
4. Life Vision Statement
5. Take Action

Tools and Practices:
- Milestone Timeline process
- Statement of Purpose
- Mind Map
- Action Plan
- SMART Goals

Level 1

Map Your Dream Life

Step 1

Follow the Mind Map Process in the *Tools of Vision* on page 211. Organize the heading of your mind map in the following way:

- Use "Life I Love" as the main center heading.

Use the following categories for the major headers:

- Family
- Health and Body
- Career
- Home
- Leisure/Hobbies
- Relationships
- Purpose
- Skills to Master

See an example of a life design mind map here:
http://erikohlsen.com/activate-your-joy-support/

Step 2

For each major heading, include major milestone goals you are setting for yourself within each category of *Step 1.*

Here are some made-up examples:

- Family Milestone: Have a truth-telling conversation with my dad or have children of my own.
- Health and Body Milestone: Stop drinking caffeine and work out three days a week consistently for a month.
- Career Milestone: Start my business and work for myself.
- Home Milestone: Plant a food garden and grow 50 percent of my food.
- Leisure/Hobbies Milestone: Join a new soccer team.

- Relationships Milestone: Have the courage to stand up for myself when I'm verbally abused by my mother.
- Purpose Milestone: Finally start the community project I've been dreaming of.
- Skills to Master: Make time to take a class in wood working so I can build my own house someday.

Level 2

Develop Short and Long Term Goals

Here you are going to use a timeline method to place your goals in a plan that makes sense to you and your current situation. Create a timeline for each milestone created in Level 1. If you want to get more detailed, create a timeline for each life category as well as the general milestone timeline.

Below is an example of what a timeline looks like. Claim your free *Activate Your Joy Life Design Game Workbook* for a full template you can use, or follow this link to see an example of a life design timeline: http://erikohlsen.com/activate-your-joy-support/

Step 1

Place *Milestones* from Level 1 on the timeline where you realistically think you can accomplish them. These are your major goals. Make sure that you place milestone goals in one-year, five-year and ten-year timeframes on your timeline at a minimum. If you are keenly focused on this process, you can add goals at whatever time intervals you want. This is ideal.

Step 2

Place all of the Skills to Master goals from your mind map on the timeline in the succession that makes the most sense to you and then move to Level 3.

Level 3

Dream Life Timeline (Reverse Engineering/Back Design)

Step 1 (only step)

Go through the timeline in detail by starting at the end of the timeline (the farthest point into the future), and working backwards (this is a reverse engineering process). You're reading the timeline in reverse from end to beginning.

Make sure that the sequencing of your goals and skills to learn make sense for what is realistic. Tweak your timeline, implementing any revelations you received during the reverse engineering process above.

Level 4

Create a Vision Statement

Create a vision statement for yourself. This is the essence of your vision integrating not only your vision but also the frame of mind statements you created in the *Transform Your Frame Mission*. A combination of your values, what makes you happy, and your life vision. The goal is to edit all this down into a two-paragraph all-encompassing statement.

Step 1

Review your written milestone goals again and describe each one in detail including:

- The skills you will need to learn
- The various stages you will reach to accomplish each milestone
- The attitude you will need to bring to it
- Include which superpowers you will need to utilize the most for each milestone goal.
- Make sure you have at least five major milestones detailed in this way

Step 2

One you have completed Step 1, read through your detailed milestones and use this to begin to write your vision statement. Look for the larger patterns behind and encompassing all your details. Check in with your motivations, needs, and frame of mind. How can you simplify all this work you have done into two four- or five-sentence paragraphs?

Step 3

Edit both the vision statement and the milestones into one document with the visions statement on top, followed by the milestones listed underneath.

Level 5

Take Action

Once you take action implementing your life design plan, life will throw its challenges at you. More like, your mind will perceive situations as challenges and you get to accept the feedback and make the needed adaptations to keep going. Remember your life design plan is only a guide and without a doubt will change and evolve.

Action Plan:

Notice how the word "action" keeps coming up in this mission? That is because "action" is the main energy needed for accomplishing goals. We are talking about action, yes, but not stressful doing. If you find yourself taking action frantically, filled with anxiety, and stressed out, then you have disconnected with your true self and gotten lost in the stories your mind is creating. Action doesn't have to mean stressful. It can be simple and joyful as well as effective.

An easy and effective way to manifest your life plan is to focus on completing the easiest and simplest tasks first. By starting with what is easiest and the most doable in the moment, you begin to check tasks off the list and you start moving toward completing your goals. Eventually, if you follow one easy task after another, you will find you have completed large bodies of work and will be ready to take on the more challenging tasks. I call this approach the easy step-by-easy-step action plan.

Step 1

You already know small easy actions you can take to implement your life plan, right? By going through this entire mission, you may have a handful of actions that you think need to be taken right away. If not, then review your timeline and reverse engineering process to see what jumps out at you. Is there a phone call you could make? A place to visit? A meeting to set up? Some research that can be done?

Write down a list of steps you can take this week. Remember that super easy steps are just fine. We tend to go for the big stuff first but all aspects of a plan will need to be met. Go ahead and start with the easiest tasks first. As you get those tasks done, go to the next easy tasks. Naturally you will begin to build a foundation to accomplish a large milestone.

If you follow this action plan, you will know when it's time to take on a milestone. You will know because everything will be in place to take on that milestone by then! It's magic!

The special sauce to this approach is simple:

- Start with the easy tasks and get them done
- Follow the path that emerges
- Anticipate and prepare for larger milestones
- Complete Large Milestone
- Repeat Easy-Step by Easy-Step Action Plan for the next milestone

Final Action

Your only real action through all of this is to trust whatever happens and stay connected with the essence of who you are. Stay present, stay true to yourself and have gratitude for the journey and your emerging pathway.

MISSION:

CULTIVATE YOUR

AWARENESS POWER

The goal of this mission is to calm your mind and awaken yourself to the present moment over and over again. Give yourself permission to find tranquility. Be at peace and stay disciplined in cultivating your awareness practices. This is so worth it.

Three Levels

1. Initiate Inner Peace
2. Moment to Moment Practice
3. Claim Awareness Power

Tools and Practices:

- Walking
- Sit Spot
- Meditation
- Body Movement (Yoga, Tai Chi, and so on)

Level 1

Initiate Inner Peace

Step 1

Choose one or two calming practices to use for this level. Walking, meditation, yoga, whatever feels right to you. See the *Tools of Connection* go to page 213 to learn more about various calming practices and what they are.

Step 2

Start by committing three times a week giving yourself twenty minutes' minimum to practice your chosen calming exercise. Put it in your calendar and set reminders if that would be helpful. Work your way up to doing a twenty-minute practice every day.

Level 2

Moment-to-Moment Calming Practice

Step 1 (one step only)

Find a timer that you can carry with you throughout the day. It can be a buzzer on a phone, a watch or some other kind of reminder device. Set a reminder to go off three times per hour. Each time during the day the reminder goes off, take ten seconds or more to stop what you are doing and focus on three calming breaths. The more you can do this moment-to-moment awareness the better.

Level 3

Claim Awareness Power

Step 1

Create a month long practice of following Level 1 and Level 2 of this mission. This time, let's make it a real challenge. Follow Level 1 and 2 for one full month.

Step 2

Once you've successfully followed levels 1 and 2 for a month or two, start adding a multiple-hour retreat. This looks like a 1-3 hour or more session of calming practices each week.

MISSION:

COMMUNICATE YOUR TRUTH

Create magic with your words and with attentive listening. You have come to a crossroads. Ready to face your fear and free yourself? Communicating your truth is difficult yet rewarding work. Your courage to accept this mission is a major investment into healthy relationships. Completing this mission has the potential to change your life forever. Make sure to take this mission level by level because you will need the practice to successfully complete the final milestone.

Three Levels
1. A Small Gesture of Truth
2. Develop a Support System and Reflect
3. Transformation Milestone

Tools and Practices:
- Attentive Listening
- Reflecting Others
- Empathetic statement
- "I" statements
- Calming Practices
- Support Team

Level 1

A Small Thorn

We all carry around small grievances we never resolve. In these cases, for many of us, it is often easier to not communicate the issues and avoid conflict. In this way, we end up stuffing our resentments down giving them time to fester.

Step 1

To build up your skills for the third level, you will want to gradually take on tough communication challenges. Start with a "small thorn" (grievance). Maybe it's something that bothers you about a relationship but it's not that big of a deal so you avoid addressing it. Choose this small issue you want to resolve with someone.

Step 2

Set up a face to face or phone meeting with the person you want to communicate with. Make sure to use your grounding and awareness tools prior to the meeting so you can show up to your conversation mindfully.

Important: Make sure you use the communication process in the Tools of Connection found on page 213 to ensure your communication meeting has the best chance for a productive process.

Level 2

Develop a Support System and Reflect

Step 1

Reflect on how Level 1 turned out. Did you follow the process? What seemed to work, where did you falter? Apply what you learned to accomplish the next level.

Step 2

In Level 3 you will take on a big communication challenge. You may want support before and after. Identify someone who can act as an accountability buddy for you. If you can't find someone, join the Activate Your Joy Facebook support group here.

https://www.facebook.com/groups/184539945414028/?source=create_flow

Level 3

Transformation Milestone

Step 1

Identify a big communication challenge. What could this be for you? Is it a truth you need to tell a family member? Heal a relationship at work? This challenge is about speaking your truth. It is not about the other person. Use the same communication process used in Level 1.

Avoid having expectations about how the other person will respond to your truth telling. Let everything play out in its own way, but ensure your own truth is shared. Remember to use "I" statements as well as empathetic statements during your communication process.

Step 2

Reflect on how Level 1 turned out. Did you follow the process? What seemed to work, where did you trip up? Check in with your support person about how the conversation turned out. Apply that learning to the next communication milestone you take on.

MISSION:

ACTIONS OF GENEROSITY

Generosity is how we create peace in our families, communities and world. In this mission you have an opportunity to spread your goodwill to others. The secret here is this—being generous is not just about others, it's about your own happiness too. The more generous you are, especially if acts of generosity are done without expectation of return, the more you generate inner joy.

Three Levels
1. A Kind Deed
2. Actions of Generosity
3. Be a Peacemaker

Tools and Practices:
- Expect nothing in return for your generosity
- Don't make the giving about your ego
- Refrain from needing a compliment or even a thank you

Suggested activities to include in your mission:
- Help a sick friend have a meal.
- Help someone move to a new home.
- Babysit a friend or family member's kids.
- Help someone with a cleaning or building project.
- Use your superpowers! Give your gift freely to others.
- Volunteer for a charity you care about.

- Give someone a ride where they need to go
- Feed the hungry
- There are so many generosity actions one can to take. Choose from this list or your own!

Level 1

A Gift of Support

Step 1

Is somebody in your life—a friend, a family member, a colleague—in need of some kind of support? What about a stranger? Helping a stranger can be a great gift of generosity as well. Choose a generosity action to take.

Step 2

Make it happen! Start with what feels achievable to you. Put the time aside and execute your generosity action.

Step 3

Check in with your feelings before, during and after. Do you feel a closer connection with this person(s) now? Do you feel good about the service you provided? Do you feel you need their love or their appreciation to feel good about what you did?

Level 2

Step Up Your Generosity Game

Step 1

Follow the Level 1 process again, although this time, plan for a larger action. What would it be? You may find you even want to plan this out ahead of time for maximum benefit.

Step 2

Make a game of taking small actions of generosity each week and a large action four times a year. You may find pure joy in this kind of work. Taking the time to plan the large actions could make a big difference in the impact, but whatever you have time and space to take on is perfect. Don't put undue pressure on yourself, otherwise you may fall into the trap of needing recognition for your generosity. Do it for the joy of it, whenever you can. In this way, you become a peacemaker for your community, spreading emotional pollen of peace and kindness.

MISSION:

FACE YOUR GRIEF

Every human carries some form of unresolved grief inside in their hearts. The grief may stem from direct experience of losing a loved one, grief of parents or grandparents passing on, or grief for the way the world is and the sad realties that happen every day on the planet. Grief itself can and does pass from generation to generation. In modern-day western culture we are not taught how to process grief. Many would rather ignore their grief than face it. They would rather not share their feelings with others and in many cases not even allow themselves to feel those feelings when they're in private.

It is not surprising many of us don't want to face our grief, and the pain and trauma that may be associated with it. As you work through this mission, be gentle with yourself. Ensure you have set up a support system to help you work through anything that comes up that is too much to process on your own. Facing your grief may be a turning point in your life where you put down some of the emotional baggage you have been carrying around. That is why this mission is so important. Let go of what doesn't serve you any longer. Be free from the grip of fear.

Four Levels
1. The Grief Altar
2. Create a Grief Ritual
3. Make an Agreement

Tools and Practices:
- Grief Altar
- Grief Ritual
- Support Team
- Music

Level 1

The Grief Altar

(An altar is usually a raised platform used to focus energy for rituals and to make offerings.)

Step 1

The idea of creating an altar is to honor the loss you are grieving and to provide a space to process this grief. Create an altar with mementos and symbols representing a major grief you feel. Use pictures, physical items, drawings, art, anything representing the person to build the altar. The altar can be on top of a dresser, a desk, or any surface you can devote to it.

Step 2

Find music that reminds you of the person, animals, place or thing. Finding music that elicits an emotional response would be good choice.

Step 3

Find a support person or persons who can be there for you when you need to talk to someone. Go to the Activate Your Joy Facebook support page for more:

https://www.facebook.com/groups/184539945414028/?source=create_flow

Level 2

Create a Grief Ritual

Step 1

Give yourself some time, at least one hour or more for this exercise. Make sure you will not be disturbed unless it is someone on your support team. Light a candle on your altar when you are ready to begin.

Step 2

Who or whatever you chose for your altar is the focus of this exercise. It can be a lost loved one, or something tragic that happened to you that you've never processed. Write down or speak out every single thing you're feeling in the space about the subject of your grief. Whatever feels natural and most comfortable. For some, speaking out loud is too awkward so write it down instead.

The more you get in touch with what you're feeling, the less power your grief will have on you in the long run. The more you allow yourself to process, the stronger this healing process will be. Now sit in front of your grief altar. Put the music on and allow yourself to feel what comes up completely. If it's emotional, do your best not to block the flow of emotions no matter how intense it gets. This is your moment for deep healing. Allow it to come as strong as it wants to.

If you feel more comfortable doing this in an environment where nobody can hear you, set up that up for yourself. It's best if you can be as loud as possible without fear of people hearing. There's no one to judge you. This is about you and your feelings. Say or write anything you want to say to this person. Anything you would want different from what happened. Say it or write it down, but be as direct as possible. No editing.

Step 3

Once you have exhausted your grief in this way, move to gratitude. Give gratitude for all the ways you've been touched by or supported by the subject of your grief ritual. Then, acceptance. Write a mantra for yourself reflects your celebration gratefulness and acceptance of this loss.

Mantra example: "I fully accept the lessons I have learned and let go of what doesn't serve me."

Keep the altar up for a few days or longer. Each day go back and sit with it some more. If there's more to express, more to cry, and more to write, give yourself the space to do. Be careful you don't fall into a trap of getting stuck in grief processing where you spiral into your stories and wallow in them. Ensure you are using your inner awareness practices and limitless thinking before you open yourself up to processing emotions of grief. Check yourself. If you feel stuck, move to a different activity, especially if that feels like the best thing to do for your mental state.

Level 3

Make an Agreement

Step 1
Look for a major take-away from the ritual. Observe the Aha revelations that surface from this process. Something you learned, something you'll say or do, a new vow you have made to yourself. Take a moment and make a vow, make an agreement.

Step 2
If desired, choose one thing from the altar and put it somewhere in your house or keep it on you. A reminder of the revelation you may have harvested from your grief ritual, or to remind you of the new agreement you have made with yourself.

MISSION:
THE GIFT OF FORGIVENESS

The *Gift of Forgiveness Mission* is an opening for you to make a major transformation in your life. It is extremely important you follow this process level by level, and step by step. It's going to take time to build up to the final level. You can do this! This is another chance to let go of limiting beliefs you may be holding on to, and another chance to generate inner peace leading to more joy in your life.

Three Levels
1. A Small Letting Go
2. The Forgiveness Letter
3. The Forgiveness Conversation

Tools and Practices:
- Attentive Listening
- Empathetic Statements
- Forgiveness Letter
- Use your Superpowers found in *Awaken Your Superpower Mission*
- Calming practices developed in *Cultivate Awareness Power Mission*

Level 1

A Small Letting Go

Step 1

Pinpoint a grievance you carry around. It can be something you have done, or something you didn't do. It can be something that was done to you by someone else.

Here are some made-up examples:

- My friend never called me back and months have now gone by. They must be mad at me.
- My coworker was mean to me the other day. They must not like me.
- My dad won't help me out with my money problems or spend any time with me and my family. He must not care about us. He doesn't love us anymore (this might be a bit large of a grievance for *Step 1*).
- I didn't get the job. I must not be good enough.

Step 2

Ask yourself these questions and write down the answers:

What do you believe about the grievance, can you know for sure this is true?

What if your belief about this issue was not true?

What would your life be like if you didn't carry this grievance around with you?

Level 2

The Forgiveness Letter

Step 1

Think of a person you have a deep held resentment or awkwardness with. Go big. Set this challenge up as a major milestone in your relationship with this person. Who do you choose?

Step 2

Now you are going to write a letter to the person you want to forgive and/or ask forgiveness from. Make sure your letter follows the below guidelines:

Include in letter:

- Express what you think and feel. Use feeling words
- Avoid using "You" statements. Use "I" statements as much as possible. Own your own feelings
- Don't project onto them, making them the perpetrator
- As much as possible, avoid being a judge in this situation
- Don't make assumptions about how the other person will react or what they are thinking
- Share empathetic statements with them
- Offer them a positive idea you wish for them
- Release them from your story
- Be compassionate to them
- Be specific
- Be solution oriented

Exclude from letter:

- Blaming language
- Interrogation with lots of questions
- Making them responsible for your feeling
- Negativity

Step 2

Once you have written this letter reread it to yourself. Revise and edit as necessary ensuring you're following the outline provided for you in step one. Be bold and authentic writing this letter.

Level 3

The Forgiveness Conversation

Step 1

Set up a phone call or face-to-face meeting with this person and mark it down in your calendar.

Step 2

Before making the call or arriving at the meeting, make sure you devote at least twenty minutes to a calming or awareness practice. Engage your Limitless Thinking and Activate your Superpowers.

Step 3

Make the call or go to the set meeting. Make sure to set up a healthy container for the forgiveness conversation. The container is the agreed-upon structure of the conversation. Make sure you follow the agreement setup from the communication process found on page 213 to set up a healthy container for the conversation.

Greet each other kindly, and read the letter exactly and completely before getting into copious conversation. Ensure you have an agreement in place to not be interrupted during the reading of the letter. Use the Communication process step by step! You will be so surprised by what happens.

MISSION:
PRACTICE OF GRATITUDE

This mission will help you connect with the abundance in your life. It's time to create your own practice of gratitude. A practice of connection and awareness. A practice of celebrating your success, acknowledging milestones reached, and being grateful for good things in your life. This practice will help change your frame of mind and activate compassion and generosity in your way of being.

Your practice of gratitude encompasses small and large aspects of your life. It could be as simple as hugging your child or appreciating a good meal. It can be as vast as recognizing the discomfort in your life and giving thanks for the lessons it teaches you. Every single moment provides an opportunity to celebrate your gratitude, giving thanks for your life and all of life.

Three Levels
1. Personal Gratitude Statement
2. Share Gratitude
3. Gratitude for Challenges

Tools and Practices:
- Gratitude Reminders
- Calming practice developed in *Cultivate Awareness Power mission*
- Breath Awareness
- Time spent in nature

Suggested activities to include in your mission:

- Use a gratitude reminder
- Practice gratitude for the beauty of nature
- Carry a gratitude stone
- Say thanks before you eat
- Connect your breath with gratitude of life
- Gratitude for your relationships
- Be gracious to others. Practice appreciation.

Level 1

Personal Gratitude Statement

Step 1

Write a list of everything you are grateful for in this moment. Review the list and look for major themes you find on your list. Start to create your gratitude statement. Start sentences with "I'm thankful for ... (fill in the blank)"

Here are some examples of what I'm grateful for:

- I'm thankful for my healthy and loving children.
- I'm thankful for my beautiful and supportive wife.
- I'm thankful for my loyal and hardworking staff.
- I'm thankful for the water which nourishes life.
- I'm thankful for the food sustaining my body.
- I'm thankful for the deep love in my heart.
- I'm thankful for all the people who have the courage to make peace in their lives and in the world.

Make your gratitude statement a minimum of five sentences. More may be better, let this be a practice of gratefulness for all you have and all you are calling in for your abundant life. Make sure the statement is short enough that you able to easily read it each day.

Step 2

For one week, start your day reading or saying your gratitude statement. Feel free to incorporate it into a calming or body healing exercise found in other missions in this book.

Step 3

Incorporate a gratitude reminder into your daily practice. Setting alarms on a phone, watch or timer can work well. If you can, set this timer to go off multiple times per hour. Each time the reminder goes off, take thirty seconds to stop what you're doing and take a couple deep breaths. Give thanks for something each time.

Level 2

Share Gratitude

Step 1

Using the same process as Level 1, create gratitude statements for people you know or for things in your life. Choose three people or things (e.g., a comfy home, a meal, and so on) you want to give appreciation too.

Step 2

Take the time to create a space to share the gratitude statements that you wrote with the people you wrote them about. If this seems difficult or silly go ahead and use language that feels comfortable to you and give appreciation and thanks in whatever way feels right to you. You can't fail at this mission.

Level 3

Gratitude for Challenges

Step 1

This is a hard level of gratitude to complete. Your goal is to find gratitude in the middle of something hard or challenging. It can be something painful, emotional, or uncomfortable. Can these challenging moments be a catalyst to bring you back to the present moment? Can they remind you of who you truly are? Can they bring you home to oneness with the universe? They can, but it will take patience and practice.

Step 2

During the challenge or painful situation, start by changing your frame. Rather than descending into limited and stressful thinking like you might do normally in this situation, look for the gem or silver lining of the moment. Acknowledge what the challenge is pushing you to do or not to do. Find the key lesson or transformative action that the challenge is leading you towards and act upon it. It will only reveal itself through your gratitude.

Step 3

Practice allowing the stress or pain of your challenges to guide your next actions. Evolve your gratitude routine to reflect these signals as they happen. This keeps you aligned with the changing environment and the changes happening inside of you.

Be grateful for the transformations that happen through this process and keep going!

MISSION:
THE NATURE OF HAPPINESS MISSION

What do you love to do? Would you be happier if you did more of this? The happiness mission is all about doing what you love. Intentionally put aside and plan time to experience your favorite things and create new, powerful routines and habits. Do something you have always dreamed of doing. Learn something you have always wanted to learn. Express your creativity and have fun!

Three Levels
1. Day of Happiness
2. Week of Joy
3. Month of Bliss

Tools and Practices:
- Play Music
- Do your art
- Play your favorite sport
- Go into Nature
- Dance
- Celebrate and share your joy with others

Level 1

Day of Happiness

Step 1

Schedule your day of happiness. Put a date on the calendar and stick to it like you would a doctor appointment, job interview or plane travel.

Step 2

Create a plan for your day of happiness. Start by making an agenda for the day including activities you enjoy. Prioritize a plan that is nurturing. Make it special. See above for suggested activities and choose your own too. Choose what you love.

Avoid: Spending lots of money, ingesting copious amounts of intoxicants or other distracting activities that may have negative side effects.

Step 3

When the day arrives put your plan into action. But ... sometimes the best plan is the one we throw away. Allow yourself to connect with your gut feeling the morning of your special day. If you feel drawn to do something spontaneously instead, give yourself that gift. Let the day take its own course if it feels right. Otherwise, follow your plan.

Enjoy your day!

Level 2

Week of Joy

Step 1

Schedule a week-long plan for your happy living. The goal of this week is to integrate activities that nurture and support your happiness within a normal week of your life. This is going to be a challenge, but stick to it and you will be rewarded for your effort.

Step 2

Prioritize at least one hour of joyful activity per day. If you are a busy person and don't feel capable of doing this, consider getting up an hour earlier each day to accomplish this mission. Spend at least one hour a day doing something that makes you happy.

Level 3

Month of Bliss

Step 1

To complete a month of bliss, you repeat Level 2 for four weeks in a row. Realistically, spending an hour every day, seven days a week in this pattern may be difficult. Give yourself a better chance of success by spending a minimum of five days a week for a month following the Week of Joy, Level 2.

Step 2

See your purpose awaken as you focus doing what you love! Take time once a week to reflect and write down what it is like to prioritize things that make you happy each day. Ask yourself if you want to make this a forever pattern in how you live life.

MISSION:
HEAL YOUR BODY MISSION

Your body deserves your love and attention. Small changes in your habits will help you take control of your own health and well-being. In this mission you will put into action a plan to heal and care for your body. A practical plan that fits your special circumstance, body type, lifestyle, and mental state. While you begin this mission, make sure to avoid judging yourself for any stories you have about what you "should" or "shouldn't" have been doing for your body. There is no shame here. Take action now to reduce your stress and nourish your body.

Three Levels
1. Gift for Your Body
2. Create a Self-Care Plan
3. Make a Commitment

Tools and Practices:
- Drink plenty of water each day
- Move throughout each day (walking, running, stretching etc.)
- Eat until you're 3/4 full
- Practice eating unprocessed foods (read ingredients and learn the difference between processed and unprocessed foods
- Practice body awareness and connections between your activities and consumption and how it makes your body feel.
- Put on your exercise clothes first thing when you wake up
- Food Journal

- Heath Trackers, Reminders

Level 1

A Small Gift for Your Body

Step 1

In this level you are going to create a self-care plan for one day. First you want to choose the day. Put it on your calendar if you need to or better yet start tomorrow!

Step 2

The night before your chosen day, create a simple plan. This plan will start first thing in the morning before anything else. By starting with a body and mind focused activity, you will set the tone for the whole day. From there you can build on the momentum you generate. Make your plan simple and achievable.

Here is what you want to include in your plan for a day:

1. Choose one activity related to food or hydration. For example: avoid eating sugar for the day or drink eight glasses of water. Refer to the suggested activities above for more inspiration.
2. Choose one movement goal. For example: two twenty-minute yoga sessions or a five mile walk or hike. Refer to the suggested activities above for more inspiration.
3. Choose one of your calming exercises from previous missions.

Step 3

Execute your plan! At the end of the day reflect on how you feel. Know that one day is only a tiny beginning to creating new healthy patterns for yourself. Move to Level 2 and start planning your extended Self-Care plan.

Level 2

The Self Care Plan

Step 1

Use a Mind Map or listing process to compile goals for your optimum self-care plan. If using a mind map, "My Healthy Body" is at the center of the map. Choose focus areas like diet, movement, weight, stress reduction, physical ability, flexibility and so on for your main areas to map out.

See a Self-Care Mind Map example here:
http://erikohlsen.com/activate-your-joy-support/

Based on the mind map, create a realistic one-year timeline for your self-care plan. Use the Timeline Tool. Be sure to include in your plan a gradual changing of patterns for each day. To make your one-year plan, look at larger milestones you want to achieve in your timeline.

Then start with a daily plan you can realistically implement. Make daily rhythms like you did for Level 1. What does an optimal day look like for you?

See a Self-Care Timeline Example here:
http://erikohlsen.com/activate-your-joy-support/

Here is what you want to include in self-care plan:

1. Make a daily rhythm like in Level 1. Each week review your plan and add new routines to the daily rhythm as you can. Be realistic, but push your edges and be disciplined. Remember not to judge yourself if you find this hard. You can always start again the next day.

2. Add major body health milestones to your timeline. Some example might be: ideal weight, ideal diet, physical abilities and athleticism goals and so on.

3. Daily movement Plan

4. Food Plan
5. Hydration Plan
6. If you suffer from a chronic illness or other ongoing issues, make sure you include milestones for moving through your healing journey of these persistent issues. For example, if you have cavities and haven't seen the dentist for years, make going to the dentist a milestone to achieve.

Step 2

Review your overall plan and make edits to it after you completed Level 2.

Level 3

A Focused Commitment

Step 1

Time to implement your full self-care plan. Make this a big commitment for yourself and commit to a one-month trial of your self-care plan. Research into how humans change patterns has revealed to me that it takes approximately three weeks to change a pattern. It may take you a bit to get your momentum going.

Step 2

After your one-month trial, review your plan again and make any needed changes. Commit the rest of the year to implementing your self-care plan! Follow the daily rhythms and work towards achieving milestones you set for yourself. Just remember to do all this with no expectations of what success should look like, and accept whatever happens.

MISSION:
TEND TO NATURE

Our ecosystems provide us with water, air, energy and food to eat. In the last few hundred years, human development has unfortunately destroyed many natural ecosystems on the planet. With a little bit of care and effort, we could repair these precious environments for future generations. Now you have a chance to give back even a little bit. Planting just one tree can make a huge difference. If everyone on Earth planted one tree it would have major implications to the health of the biosphere of planet Earth.

Growing your own food is a great way to have a direct connection to nature. Growing your own food provides you with the healthiest food possible while reducing dependence on food transportation thus reducing fossil fuel consumption.

What if you could do this work in a community setting! That is even more fun and joyful. Follow this mission and contribute your energy to tend to nature and build your community. You may find yourself feeling more connected with your community and environment than ever before.

Three Levels
1. Plant a Tree and/or Spend Time in Nature
2. Grow Your Own Food
3. Plan a Community Project

Tools and Practices:

- Tree planting best practices found in *Tools of Regeneration*
- Keep it organic (Zero use of chemicals)
- Use compost teas (learn more about this in *Tools of Regeneration*, found on page 219)
- Planting bed preparation found in *Tools of Regeneration*

Level 1

Plant a Tree /Spend Time in Nature

Step 1

Choose a tree and a location. Make sure the tree is appropriate for the soils and climate where it is being planted. Make sure it will have its water needs met in the location you choose. An edible tree is suggested but choose any tree fitting the above description.

Step 2

Plan the day and plant your tree. Follow the *Tree-Planting Guide* in the *Tools of Regeneration* found on page 219. Make sure you have all the materials you need to compete the project on the day you plant your tree. Follow the *Tree-Planting Guide*!

Step 3

After your tree-planting day, follow up on your tree to make sure it has all it needs to grow and thrive. It is advisable to return one week later to make sure the tree hasn't sunk or something else happen to it. After that, visit a month later again to check. Periodically check on your tree for an entire year's cycle to make sure it is being well maintained and thriving.

Step 4

If you are unable to participate in the above steps for some reason, that is okay. Instead plan a two-hour minimum jaunt into nature. It can be a local park, a lake, a hiking trail, a mountaintop, the beach, whatever is accessible to you. Take this time to observe the nature you visit, maybe even participate in a sit spot experience. Sit spots are an incredible practice for connecting with nature and yourself (find out what a sit spot is on page 219). Look at the birds, the plants, insects and any life you see there. Reflect on how you feel being aware in nature.

Level 2

Grow Your Own Food

Step 1

Choose edible plants to grow and a good location. Unless you are already experienced at growing your own food, start small with one garden bed approximately three to four feet wide and six to eight feet long.

Step 2

Prep the garden bed following the *Garden Bed Preparation Guide* in the *Tools Regeneration* found on page 219.

Step 3

Plant your food garden! Follow best practices, whether you are planting by seed or with already sprouted plant starts. Make sure you stay dedicated to the full cycles of caring for your food garden all the way through the seasons. Learn about and harvest the food when it is ready.

Take it a step further and allow a few plants to go to seed and complete their cycle. Harvest, clean and store these seeds to grow next year.

Level 3

Plan a Community Project

Step 1

Choose a project in the community that has some element of caring for the environment. Depending on your ambition for this mission, either join an existing effort being implemented by an organization already in your community or initiate your own endeavor.

Step 2

Dedicate a set amount of time each week to the project. Make sure to be realistic with your time and what you can accomplish.

Step 3

Commit to the project until either a major milestone has been completed, a minimum of three months has gone by, or when you feel it is time to move on. Relish in the accomplishment of working with community while tending to the nature around you.

TOOLS OF VISION

Mind Mapping Tool

Mind mapping is a potent tool for brainstorming and organizing ideas.

Step 1

Pull out a large sheet of paper or use a mind mapping computer program.

Step 2

Put one circle in the center of the page. Write the main topic in here. It is the main topic of whatever you are brainstorming about. It can be at any scale. When in visioning mode you can put "LIFE" in the center of the circle.

Step 3

Brainstorm sections off of the main topic and make more circles with lines connecting them to the main topic circle. Continue until this feels exhausted.

Step 4

Off each sub-circle, create more branches, each time drilling down into more and more detail. The result will be a messy yet organized brainstorm of your ideas. Connect and combine elements that seem similar or the same worded differently.

Step 5

Continue editing and combining elements into your goals setting, statement of purpose, and other aspects of your vision.

Vision Statement:

Your vision statement, or statement of purpose is a one to two paragraph statement, which encapsulates your distilled vision for your life. This statement can be generated from your Mind Map process.

Smart Goals:

Utilize this version of SMART goals when visioning your short and long-term goals.

S pecific

M eaningful

A ction-oriented

R ealistic

T imebased

TOOLS OF CONNECTION

"What I believe about me is my business,
What you believe about me is yours."
—Byron Katie

Communication Strategy

Communication, a process of exchange, is something we do every day of our lives. Even when we are alone, we still communicate with our own mind and the environment around us. We even communicate with the sun, the wind, and the moon. Communication is an act of sacredness. We can use communication to heal our relationships, our communities and make peace on our Earth. Each of us retains these abilities innately in our living beings. Yet, some of us still find ourselves lost. Unable to cope with the turmoil of emotions we ignite in each other through our broken communication processes.

Below is a simple communication methodology. When I first put this in action I was amazed at the results. Make sure when you use this system to *always* follow the *exact* order of speaking and reflecting.

When You Are Speaking

Step 1

Setup a time to have the conversation you want to have with someone.

Step 2

Make agreements: once the space for the conversation is made, start by making an agreement. The agreement is an outline for the conversation.

Agreement 1: You must reflect the other person before you take your turn to speak, and vice versa.

Agreement 2: The person who is speaking must use "I" statements when talking about feelings. Own your own feelings.

Agreement 3: No use of insults or name-calling is allowed.

Add any additional agreements you feel are needed for a productive conversation.

Step 3

Once the agreements have been made, use the below process when you are ready to start sharing.

When

When it's your turn to speak or if you're the first to speak start with the "when." This is identifying the thing that happened. It might be something like "When you didn't call at the time you were going to be home, I felt worried," "When you slammed the door ..." "When you called me a ..."

Make sure to only state the facts and don't add insults or make assumptions, "I was angry; I knew you weren't going to call, you're so mean ... you're so lazy ..." or anything like that. Keep it to the facts, clear and simple. Then move to "I think."

I Think

At this point you want to state the thoughts you went through in your mind when the issue happened. Again, don't pass judgment on the thoughts or put blame on the other person. Only share what you thought. "I thought, 'I wonder why he didn't call me? I hope he's okay.' " Or maybe, "I thought, wow she is mad."

Then move to the feeling words.

I Feel

The feeling phase is about sharing the emotions you felt. Whatever those emotions are, validate them and be authentic with yourself. Again, do your best not to cast blame or judgment on the other person. Your feelings are yours and yours alone. In fact, this whole sharing of your feelings is your story of what you thought happened, and how you felt. It doesn't mean it is or isn't true. You might say, "I felt scared you didn't call, and frustrated because I didn't know what you were actually doing or where you were."

When you're listening

Reflection: the listener must always do this before responding with their story! Reflecting during the communication protocol is the pillar of its success.

Step 1: Clarifying questions

When you are in the listening role and the other person has finished, you want to first start with clarifying questions and ask if there's more.

The process of asking if there's more and asking clarifying questions allows the speaker to fully share whatever is going on. Sometimes it takes a little bit more than the initial sharing to get it all out. Clarifying questions are helpful because you may have misinterpreted something right off the bat and asking for clarification might solve some of the emotional charge that can come up in the conversation.

Step 2

When you're the person reflecting, you want to reflect the things the other person has said without translating it into your own emotional viewpoint. If you felt triggered or attacked during the other person's talking time, the reflection and clarifying time is **not** the time to share those feelings. It's more important to reflect using the exact words shared with you, rather than what you translated in your head.

Step 3: Empathy statement

(An Empathy statement is a statement which validates what another person is feeling. They allow the speaker to know their feelings are acceptable and understood.)

When you're reflecting, make sure to start with an empathetic statement so the other person knows you heard them and you have compassion for them. This will go a long way toward resolving the conflict and creating an atmosphere where you'll be heard. Once you have fully reflected, clarified, and confirmed your empathy, it's your turn to speak and follow the same exact protocol with the roles reversed.

Keep these best practices in mind!

Not responding

When you are in the listening role, it is not your job to respond while the other person is sharing until you have reflected completely and it is your turn to speak.

Practice attentive listening and use your awareness skills. Catch yourself if you find yourself getting lost in your own thoughts of what you want to say and end up missing what the other person is sharing.

Not attacking

When it's your turn to communicate make sure you are not putting blame on the other person. Use "I" statements rather than "You" statements. Do your best not to make assumptions. Stay open to discovering that things may not be what you think they are.

Create space for the other person to speak authentically in the conversation. If you attack and put blame, then likely you'll get a retaliatory defensive response. This is hugely important for this communication process to work! Stay aware! Stay grounded! Do your best. Forgive yourself if it takes you time to learn how to do this!

AWARENESS PRACTICES

Sit Spots:

A sit spot is an effective way to calm your body and mind towards finding a sense of inner peace. This tool is used extensively in nature awareness schools and has been an important tool for thousands of years for indigenous cultures.

Find a place in nature. If you live in an urban environment, it can even be on your front porch, a park in the city, anywhere outside and convenient to go to every day.

The basic sit spot practice requires you to sit in your spot for a minimum of twenty-five minutes. During this time, you drop into inner and outer awareness. Be prepared to fuss for a while as your mind and body find a way to rest and relax. This is normal and to be expected. This is a special time to practice being fully present. Activate all your senses to notice the patterns all around you. Be especially aware of animals and their movements. Often it takes a minimum of twenty minutes for wildlife to relax and come back, once disturbed by you or another. Listen intently to the sounds of birds, the movements of insects and animals. Pay attention to the patterns of vegetation and the interaction and relationships between things.

Meditation:

For thousands of years, meditation has proven to be one of the most effective calming practices. There are thousands of different ways to meditate. Many guided meditation systems are available for those that seek it out.

Music:

Listening and playing music can be one of the most joyful of activities for calming your inner voice. These activities engage the right side (creative side) of the brain and take over mental functioning. Often when a person gets into "the groove" with their music, they enter an emotional state devoid of obsessive thinking and grounded in present moment awareness.

Sports:

If you are into sports, that could be a great asset to your inner peace. Playing sports often takes a strong sense of present moment awareness. Thinking subsides and moment-to-moment actions take over. Utilize your love of sports to generate a strong sense of awareness.

Being in Nature:

Spending time in nature—walking, camping and so on—can provide an incredible opportunity to feel into your awareness. Daily walks can offer an excellent way to be in nature on a daily basis and give yourself some space each day to ground yourself in awareness of present moment.

Yoga, Tai Chi, Other:

Yoga, Tai Chi and other body-to-mind connection practices are extremely powerful in generating inner peace and awareness.

TOOLS OF REGENERATION

Self-Care and Body-Care Tools

- Food Journal: create a food journal and track what you eat.
- Find a diet that is right and healthy for you and stick to it.
- Use a Health Tracker, such as Fitbit, Health Apps, Spire, other trackers.
- Utilize online or in-person exercise trainings.
- Engage a health care practitioner or professional you can build trust with.
- Utilize your limitless thinking.
- Start a movement practice, yoga, Tai Chi, bike riding, hiking and so on.

TEND TO NATURE TOOLS

Tree Planting Guide

Step 1: Digging and prepping the hole

Dig the hole at least twice the size of the roots or pot of the tree you're planting. When you dig your hole, make sure the soil that comes out of the hole is placed nearby and protected from being stepped on or compacted during the digging process.

Pro tip: I like to use a wheelbarrow or a large pot to put the soil in as I dig my hole. This makes it easier to pour the soil back around the tree when I'm ready.

If the soil you dig in is thick clay, you may want to dig a square hole rather than a round hole. A round hole dug in thick clay may result in the tree's roots spinning around the circular clay surface once they grow out that far. A square hole will give corners and edges for roots to stick into.

If you are planting your tree in a hot season and the ground is extremely dry, make sure to fill the hole with water and let the water soak in prior to planting your tree. If possible, research best timing practices for planting your tree in your climate.

Make sure you have compost or aged manure on hand to plant with the tree. It is also advised to have some kind of mulch material like wood chips, straw, leaves or some other non-toxic, biodegradable material.

Step 2: Planting the Tree

Place the tree in the hole you have made with the roots down. Make sure to check the depth of your hole compared to the length of your tree roots. If you've dug a hole that's too deep, fill it up with soil to match the length of the tree roots or tree pot.

Plant your tree and backfill around the roots with roughly half compost and half native soil. Again, make sure the trees are not too deep and gently adjust the root ball upwards if the tree starts to sink. Compress air pockets as you backfill around the roots.

Pro tip: to really give your tree an incredible start, sprinkle some Mycorrhizae fungi inoculant on the roots of the tree before planting. These fungi have a symbiotic relationship with 90 percent of the worlds plants. They grow on the roots of the plants and trees, feeding them nutrients from the surrounding soil.

Pro tip: if you're planting a bare-root fruit tree, start by planting the tree a little deeper and slowly pull the tree up to ensure its roots are pointed downward. Make sure to compress any air pockets out of the hole so the tree doesn't sink later. Fruit trees generally like to have their root crown just above or at the same level as the natural grade. Make sure that the graft union on grafted trees is pointed away from strong prevailing winds and sun (i.e. in the Northern hemisphere we point our graft wounds north or northeast away from the southern sun and westerly breezes).

Step 3: Water in the Tree

Water in your tree. Look to see if the tree sinks and add more soil or gently pull up on the ball if the tree sinks or the soil sinks after the first watering.

Pro tip: water your tree in with an aerated compost tea. Aerated compost tea is a diverse mixture of either bacterial or fungal dominated compost, which bubbles under air pumps for twenty-four to thirty-six hours. It is one of the best ways to inoculate your soil with beneficial organisms, increasing the health and vitality of your plantings. See below to learn more.

Step 4: Mulching

Once the tree has been planted and watered in, put more compost on the surface of the soil around the tree (approximately one inch). On top of the compost put your mulch (e.g. wood chips, leaves, straw), approximately between two and four inches or more. Make sure not to cover the trunk of the tree with compost or mulch. Keep the mulch at least ten inches away from the trunk.

Make sure the root crown at the trunk of the tree is exposed and at or slightly above the natural grade.

Step 5: Watering Plan

Make sure your tree will have the water it needs to survive. If planting in an arid or drought-prone environment, ensure your tree has adequate irrigation.

Planting Bed Preparation Guide:

Step 1: Choose a Location

Choose a location for your planting bed. If growing vegetables or other annual plants (plants that only grow for only one year), choose a location that is both close to your house and in the sun as much as possible.

Step 2: Clean up the Area

If the area is covered in vegetation you may want to mow it prior to prepping the bed. If the area has other materials on it, make sure to do a good cleanup before prepping your bed.

Step 3: Layout

Measure out your bed. For the *Tend to Nature Mission* choose a minimum size of three to four feet wide and six to eight feet long for your planting bed. Make sure you have adequate room around the bed to walk for planting and harvesting without stepping in the bed.

Step 4: Loosen Soil

Loosen all the soil in your bed using a broad fork or a hand fork. If the soil is extremely dry and compacted, water it in gently over the period of a couple days before digging. In some situations, machinery may be appropriate to use in loosening the soil. Try to do it by hand first if you can.

As you loosen the soil, be careful not to step on and compact the areas you've already loosened. Loose, well-aerated soil is a key condition for growing most edible plants.

Step 5: Adding Compost

Add compost or composted manure to the bed. Use a hand fork to move that compost or material in. After you have integrated your compost into your bed, add another one-inch layer over the surface of your bed. If you have followed the instructions correctly, your planting bed should be slightly raised above the natural grade around it due to your loosening and adding of compost. This is a good sign!

Step 6: Choosing Plants and Planting

Hopefully by now you have chosen the plants you want to plant here. I suggest starting with easy to grow annual vegetables if this is your first time. Lettuce, tomatoes, squash, and edible greens are all fairly easy to grow in most climates. If you are in a wet and not so sunny climate, tomatoes may not be a good fit. Choose plants you know to grow well in your area by asking locals in your region.

When you plant your plants, plant them at the suggested spacing and try not to overly compact the garden bed during planting.

Step 7: Watering

Water your plants in thoroughly after planting. Make sure your garden bed has adequate water for a thriving and stress free garden throughout the year. If needed, install an irrigation system or water by hand daily or every other day.

Step 8: Maintenance and Harvesting

Don't forget about your garden! Food gardens do require maintenance and tending. Visit your garden often (if you located it near your house, hopefully you will be visiting without effort), and care for it using your common sense. Do your own research more to learn about best practices for harvesting and eating the food you grow.

Pro-Tip: Aerated Compost Teas

These homemade, liquid fertilizers and inoculants are changing the face of landscaping. Utilizing worm castings, mature compost, and other ingredients, compost teas grow beneficial bacteria and fungi in an aerated liquid environment. Often brewed with an air-pump-injected container (of varying sizes) for twenty-four to thirty-six hours, the resulting biological inoculant can be sprayed directly on the soil or in some cases, the leaves of plants.

ACKNOWLEDGMENTS

First and foremost, I must acknowledge my amazingly loving wife, Lauren Ohlsen. She has been there for me during many of the vulnerable stories I share in this book. Always the caretaker, always supportive, keeping me on a good path. She's my supercharged accountability buddy and the most amazing mom our kids could ever hope for. Thank you!

Thank you to my two incredible children, Phoenix and Iyla. Your encouragement, inspiration, understanding, and love have fed my soul in ways I can hardly write with words. I am the luckiest dad in the universe.

I want to thank my siblings, Gina, Mary and Pete. When you read many of my stories, I think you know what I'm talking about. Thanks for being there with me through it all and supporting this sharing of some of your story.

Thank you to my beta readers, Damien and Javan. You were the first people to read my book and I was pretty scared to give it to you. Thank you for taking the time and for all of your great and important feedback that helped make this book a success.

Thank you to my editor, Spencer Borup. After working with other editors on my children's books I was pretty scared to receive your feedback on *Activate Your Joy*. Thank you for making the editing process so pleasant!

Thank you to my amazing launch team who has made this book a success. Special thanks to Joseph for your incredible proof reading skills at such a crucial time in the production of this book.

Last but not least I want to thank the entire Self-Publishing School community, and my writing/publishing coach Ramy Vance. I never could have accomplished this book without your program and all your support.

If anyone reading this has aspirations to write a book, I could not refer you strong enough to the Self-Publishing School. Learn more about this fantastic program here:

https://xe172.isrefer.com/go/sps4fta-vts/bookbrosinc1941